MW00803528

Healthy 80/10/10
RAW VEGAN
RECIPES

By Louise Koch

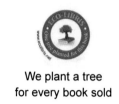

We plant a tree
for every book sold

isbn: 978-8792632-67-8

Photos: Louise Koch

Portrait: Stephan Arnskov, BHP foto

Graphic design: Louise Koch

 Published by Mill House publishers, Denmark
www.millhouse-publishers.com

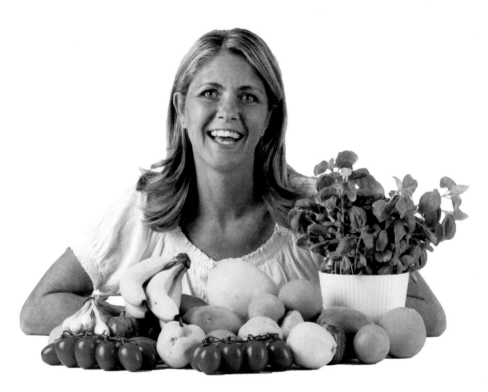

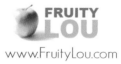

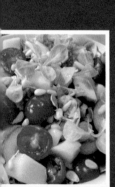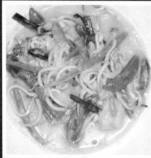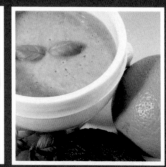

Healthy 80/10/10
RAW VEGAN
RECIPES

By Louise Koch

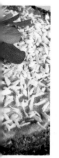
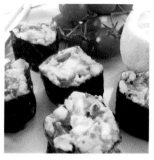
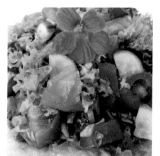
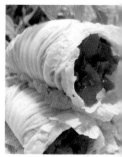

RECIPES

LOW FAT:

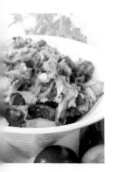
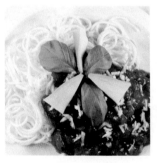
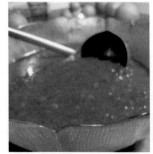
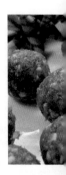

MEDIUM FAT:

 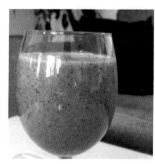 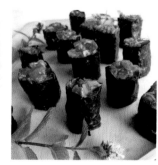 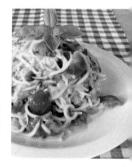

HIGH FAT:

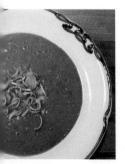
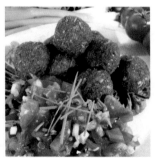
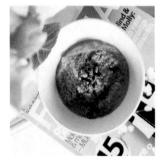
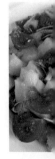

JUICES & SMOOTHIES:

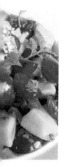
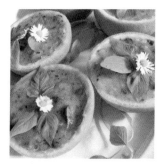
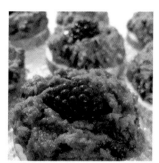
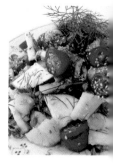

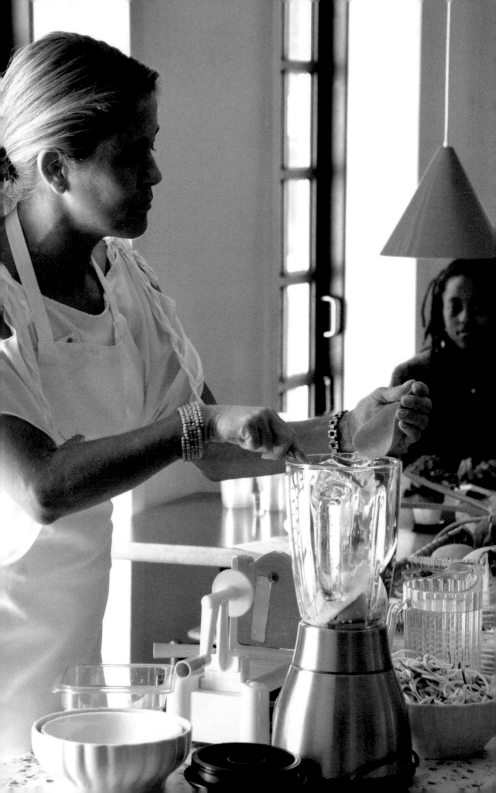

GET HEALTHY!

Would you like to be truly healthy? Now you have the chance. This recipe book will give you some amazing raw food recipes made from raw fruits and vegetables. They are easy, simple and super nutritious and your body will simply love it.

ABOUT LOUISE

My name is Louise Koch, I'm Danish and back in 2009 I was very ill. Nothing worked properly: my liver didn't function; I had severe adrenal fatigue; gout; insomnia; candida; very low hormone production; I had daily anxiety attacks for 7 years and a doctor told me that I had so much damage to my cells and DNA that the next step would be cancer if I did not do something radical. So I searched for a way out trying all the conventional and alternative treatments I could find. Unfortunately nothing worked until I came across a raw food diet called the 80/10/10 diet. Over the course of one month I slowly began to eat more and more raw foods and primarily fruit. I removed all overt fats from my diet so my blood sugar would be stable when I started to eat high amounts of fruit and then a couple of weeks later I was ready to do the diet full on. I ate mostly what is called 'mono-meals' (only one type of fruit in each meal), green smoothies and salads with soft vegetables. Step by step I rebuilt my body with the healthiest food on the planet, so that my body had the energy to heal itself. Every now and then I also made some more creative dishes like cakes, soups and nori rolls and these are among the recipes you will find in this book.

After one to two years on the diet all my ailments disappeared and today I'm perfectly well again. Before I became ill I had worked as a television producer for 10 years but I decided to skip the stressful lifestyle and instead I began to help other people get well naturally. So today I am an author, speaker, coach and event planner with the sole purpose of helping other people to get healthy and happy. The strategy I used to get well again was not only a diet change but also a lifestyle change and the adaptation of a new mental outlook. If you want to learn more about my story and the natural way of healing that I have found, please visit my webpage at www.fruitylou.com

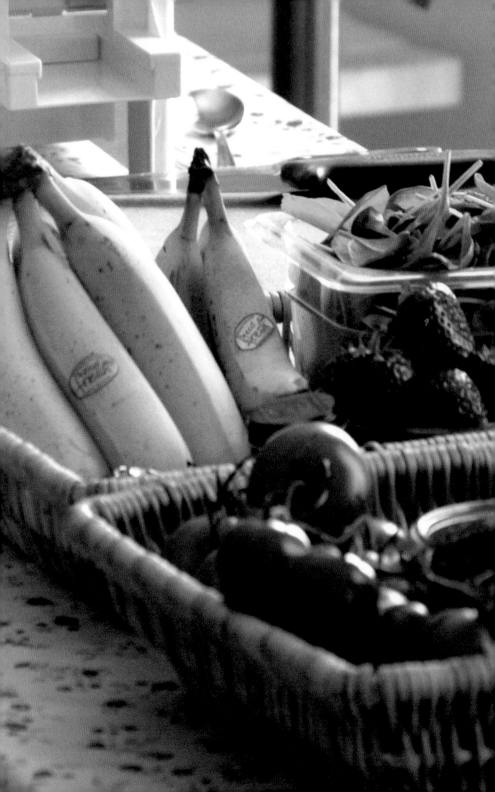

THE RECIPES

The recipes in this book are not a true representation of what you would expect to find in the 80/10/10 diet because the diet doesn't actually require you to make any recipes. Instead you simply eat the fruits and vegetables the way they are - fresh, raw and ripe, straight from nature. But I have created some recipes for people who enjoy making recipes. Most of the recipes in this book are very simple and what I would call every-day recipes, while others are a little more complex and intended for occasional treats. Therefore you should use this book only as a supplement if you want to follow the basic 80/10/10 raw food diet. But what is this 80/10/10 diet all about you may ask? Here are some explanations.

RAW FOODS

"Raw food" means that you do not heat your food but eat it in its raw state. You do not cook your food by boiling, roasting, grilling, steaming, baking or heating it in any way. To eat raw foods is not a new phenomenon, because we did it before we invented fire and in fact, today humans are the only species on this planet to heat their food in order to eat it. All other species eat it the way it is found in nature - whole, fresh, raw and ripe.

80/10/10

There are several schools of thought within the raw food movement and the two most known, are "*Gourmet raw food*" and "*80/10/10*". They are very different from each other and this recipe book is focused on the **80/10/10** principles as explained by **Doug Graham**. The percentages stand for **"minimum 80% carbohydrates, maximum 10% protein and maximum 10% fat"** of your daily calorie intake. 80/10/10 is a diet very low in fat, which means that you mainly eat fruit, some vegetables and leafy greens plus very small amounts of overt fat (e.g. avocados, coconut, seeds and nuts). It is the most natural and simple of all the dietary schools and almost the opposite to Gourmet raw foods. Gourmet raw food uses refined sugars, salt, oils, syrups, cocoa powder, super foods plus large amounts of nuts, seeds and oils. They also sometimes heat the food up to 42 degrees and use a dehydrator, whereas the 80/10/10 diet strives to use primarily whole, fresh, raw, ripe and organic produce and the keyword is 'simple' with a minimum of processing and alteration. The raw version of the 80/10/10 diet is also known as **HCLF (High Carb Low Fat) or LFRV (Low Fat Raw Vegan).**

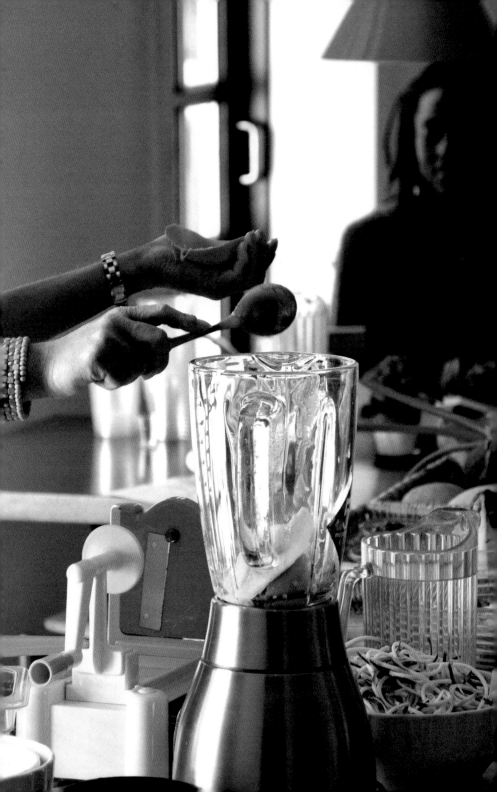

BEFORE YOU BEGIN...

Before you start there are a few things you need to know. First of all it is important that you keep to the 80/10/10 principles if you want to use a fully raw diet to improve your health. To help you in this I have divided the recipes into the four following categories: Low fat, Medium fat, High fat and Juices & smoothies. You can eat the recipes with low fat as often as you please but you should only eat the high fat recipes on special occasions and not every day. Otherwise you may get too much fat which can potentially destablize your blood sugar levels. A good way to keep track of the percentages is to use an online program like www.cronometer.com - at least for the first week.

THE PORTIONS
All the recipes are made for one person only but they ar not necessary large enough to give you the calories you need for a meal. The recipes can also be used just as a snack or a starter and you should always make sure you are getting enough calories in each meal by using an app or an online program like www.cronometer.com.

FOOD COMBINING
The dishes have been made so that they taste good and do not necessarily comply with common food combining guidelines. If you have digestive issues you may want to re-search a little about food combinations and I can recommend you try to eat more simple meals and mono meals (only one type of fruit in each meal).

GARLIC AND CHILLI
Some of the recipes have the option to add garlic or chilli but I only recommend it if you are quite healthy. Both garlic and chilli will irritate your body and your body will try to expel it quickly. If this happens you will notice your eyes and nose start to run as well as your sweat smells bad. If you are ill it is not helpful to give your body any extra burdens, so try to stay on a pretty clean diet.

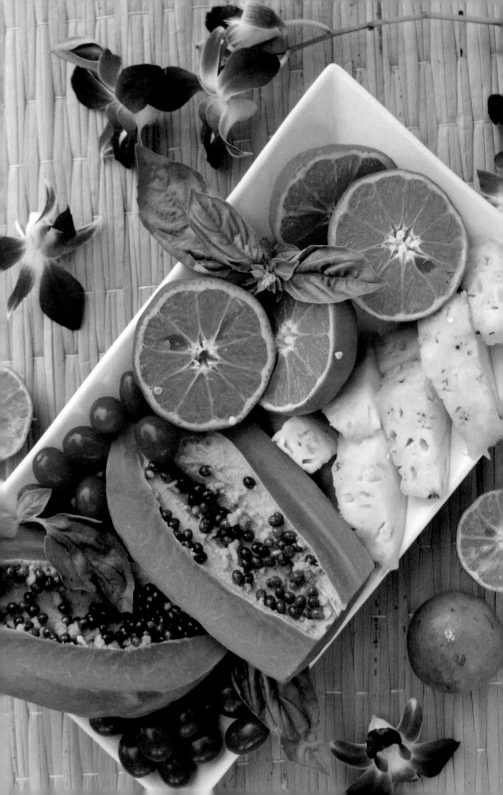

TOOLS

At the lower edge of each recipe you will find some purple symbols that indicate which tools you will need for the recipe. For example: a food processor, a spiralizer (or Julienne peeler), a bamboo mat, a citrus press/ juicer or a coffee grinder. Some basic things you will most likely also need are a chopping board, a good knife, a bowl, a plate, a glass and a spoon. The best thing is that you don't need any pots and pans for cooking and therefore you should have considerably less dishes to wash up than you would after a cooked meal.

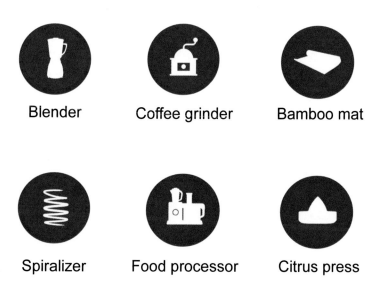

Blender	Coffee grinder	Bamboo mat
Spiralizer	Food processor	Citrus press

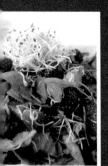 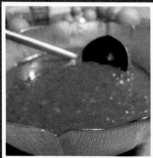 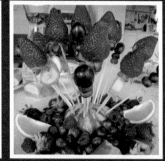 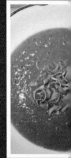

LOW

Recipes with low fat

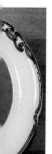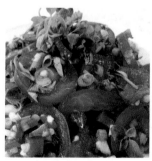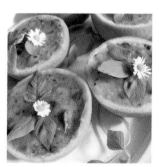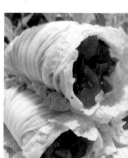

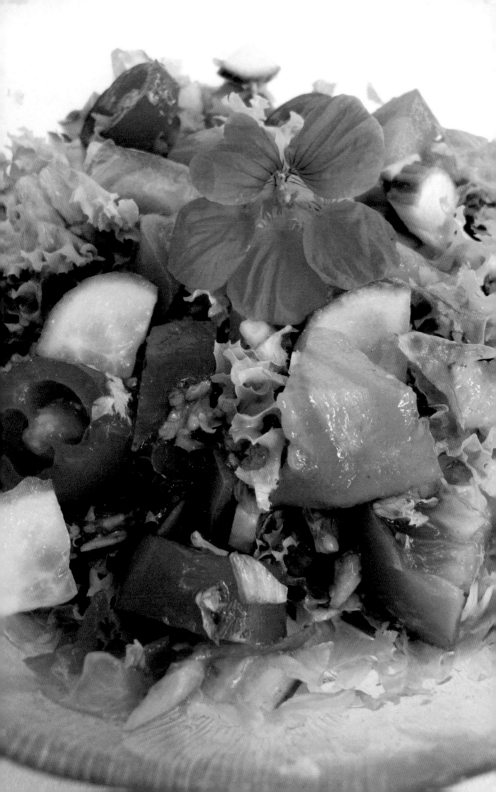

PERSIMMON SALAD
With Orange Juice

- 1/2 cucumber
- 8 plum tomatoes
- 4 persimmons or 1 papaya
- 1/2 head of Lollo Bionda lettuce
- The juice from 1 orange

Cut the cucumber into slices and then into quarters. Halve the tomatoes and cut the persimmons into smaller pieces. Slice the lettuce into strips and mix everything well in a bowl. Squeeze the juice from an orange over the salad as a dressing.

Alternatively, if you want to use papaya instead of persimmon, prepare as follows: Cut the papaya in half lengthwise and remove the seeds. Use the tip of a knife to slice diagonal lines in both directions so that you crosshatch little square dice. Use a spoon to loosen the dice from the papaya skin and add them to the salad.

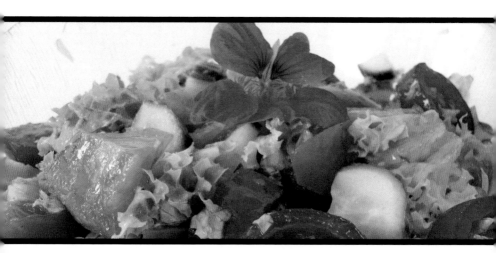

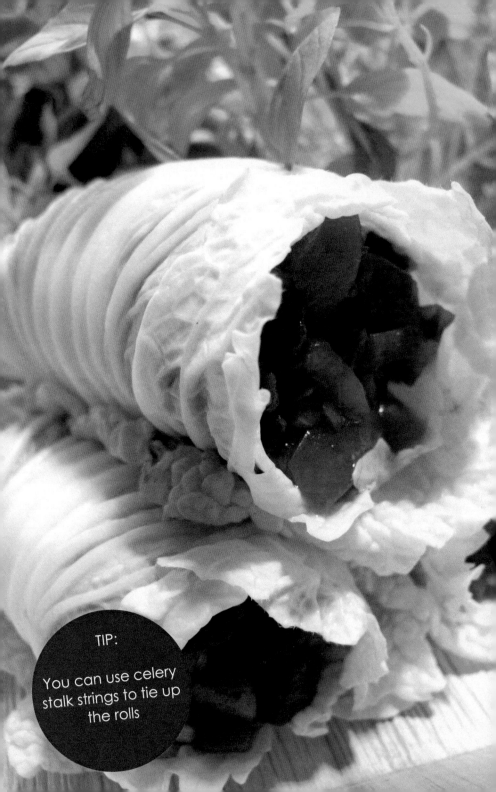

TIP:

You can use celery stalk strings to tie up the rolls

CHINESE ROLLS
With Thai Basil

- 6 medium cherry tomatoes
- 2 spring onions
- 1 red bell pepper
- 1 green bell pepper
- 2 sun dried tomatoes
- 6 large dates
- 1 handful of Thai basil
- 1 head of Chinese cabbage

Chop everything, except the cabbage, into smaller pieces and place them in a bowl. Mix well so that the dates make it all stick together.

Spread out the cabbage leaves on a chopping board and place one spoonful of the filling on the thick end of each leaf. Roll up the leaves and place the rolls on a platter. Serve and enjoy.

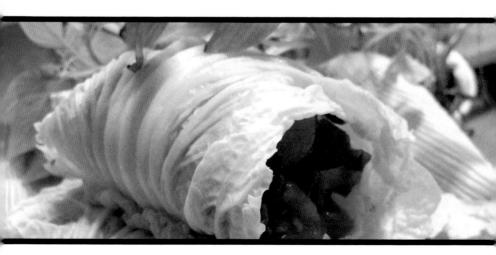

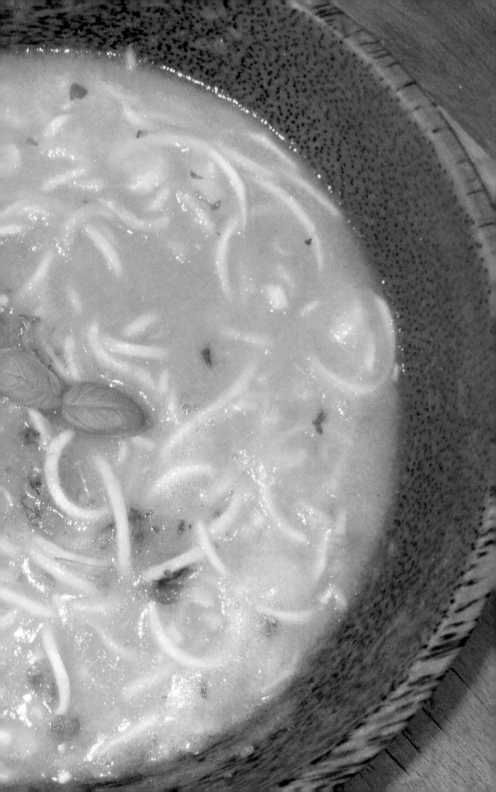

ORANGE NOODLES
With Spring Onions

- 1 zucchini
- 5-7 mandarins
- 1/2 honeydew melon
- 1 spring onions
- 1 handful of beansprouts
- 3-4 baby corn
- 1/2 lemon
- Some fresh thyme
- Optional: 1/2 clove of garlic

Blend the mandarin, the honeydew melon and the juice of the lemon together in a blender (without the seeds and skin of course). If you are well enough you can add some garlic. Blend everything into a fine soup and pour into a bowl. Chop up the spring onion and the baby corn. Add them to the soup along with the bean sprouts and some roughly chopped thyme. Finally use a spiralizer or a Julienne peeler to make noodles from the zucchini. Add the noodles to the soup and stir in well.

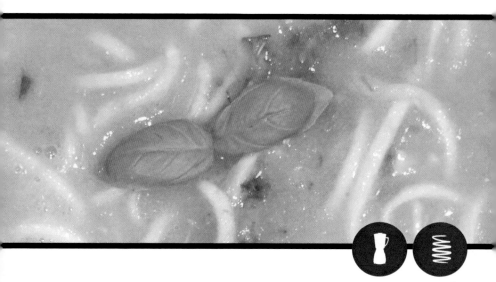

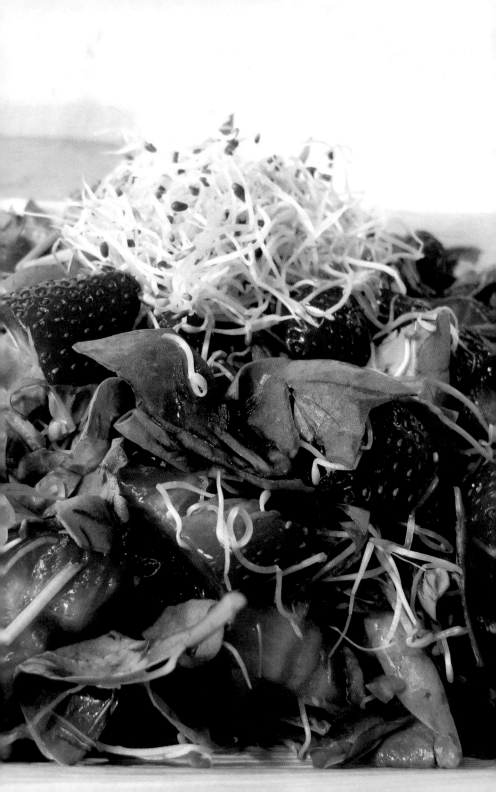

STRAWBERRY SALAD
With Mango-Basil Dressing

Salad:
- 70 gr baby spinach
- 400 gr of strawberries
- 40 gr alfalfa sprouts

Dressing:
- 1 mango
- 1 handful of basil
- 1 1/2 dl water

The salad:

Rinse the baby spinach and the strawberries well and chop them into smaller pieces (if the strawberries are organic you can eat the green calix too). Mix everything together and add the alfalfa sprouts but make sure to keep some back for decoration.

The dressing:

Blend the mango, basil and water into a delicious dressing. Place the mixed salad on a plate and poor the dressing over. Decorate or garnish with alfalfa sprouts on top.

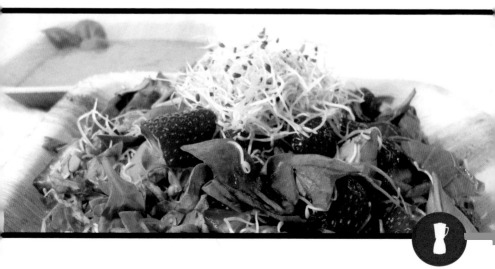

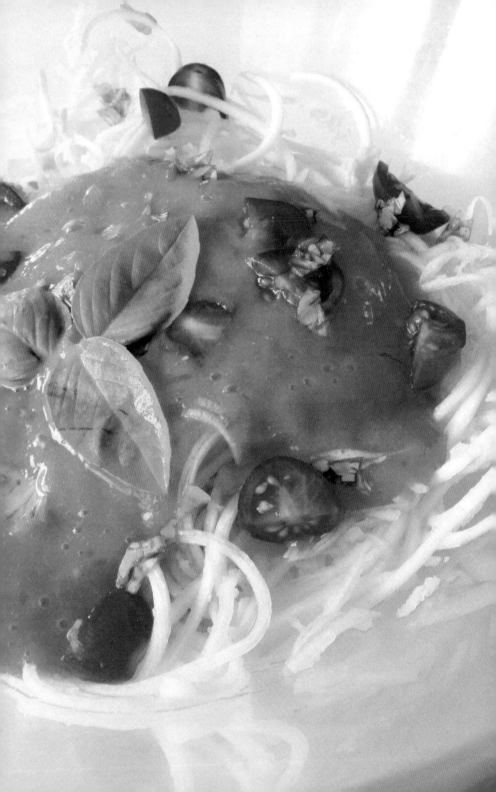

MANGO NOODLES
With Tomatoes and Spring Onions

- 1 large mango
- 1 large zucchini
- 14 cherry tomatoes
- 10 leaves of fresh basil
- 1 spring onion
- Optional: 1/2 a clove of garlic

Using a spiralizer or a Julienne peeler, cut the zucchini into long slim noodles. Place them in a large bowl. Put the 'fruit pulp' of the mango (not the pit) in the blender along with the spring onion and 8 of the cherry tomatoes (optional: add the garlic to taste, if you are very healthy). Blend everything into a creamy dressing and poor it on top of the zucchini pasta. Cut the rest of the cherry tomatoes into quarters and roughly chop the basil. Sprinkle tomatoes and basil on top of the pasta and serve.

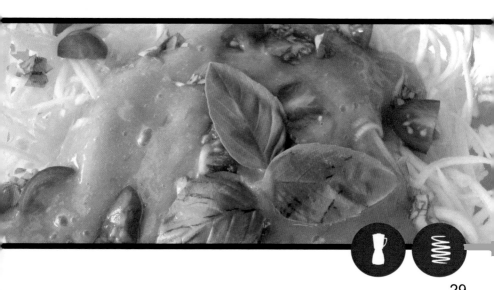

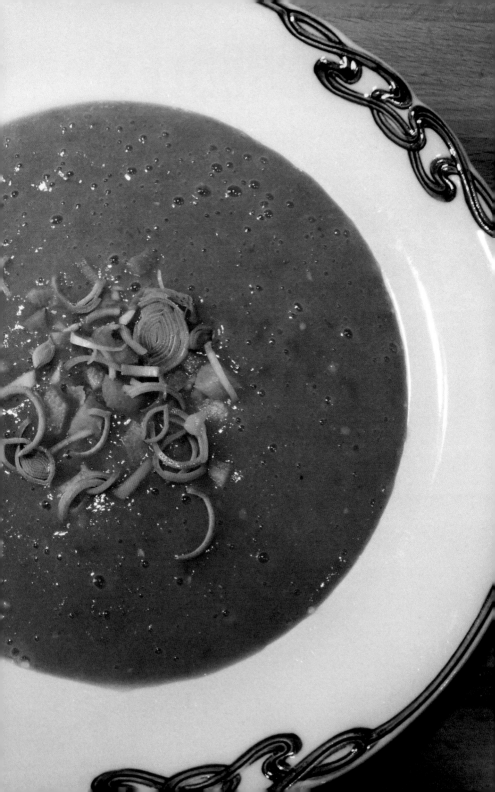

TOMATO SOUP
With Ramsons

- 6 large tomatoes
- 5 cherry tomatoes
- 1 mango
- 1 leek
- 3-6 ramsons leaves
- 1 sun dried tomato
- 1 carrot
- 6 leaves of fresh basil
- 3 long chives
- A little bit of water

Peel the mango and remove the fruit pulp from the pit. Blend the mango with the tomatoes, the leek (save some for decoration), the sun dried tomato, the chives, the basil, half of the carrot plus the ramsons. Add a little bit of water and blend at high-speed until you get a thick creamy soup. Add more water if needed. Cut the rest of the carrot into fine chunks and slice the rest of the leek thinly. Garnish the soup with the carrot and slices of leek.

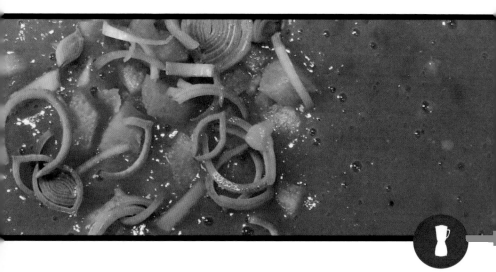

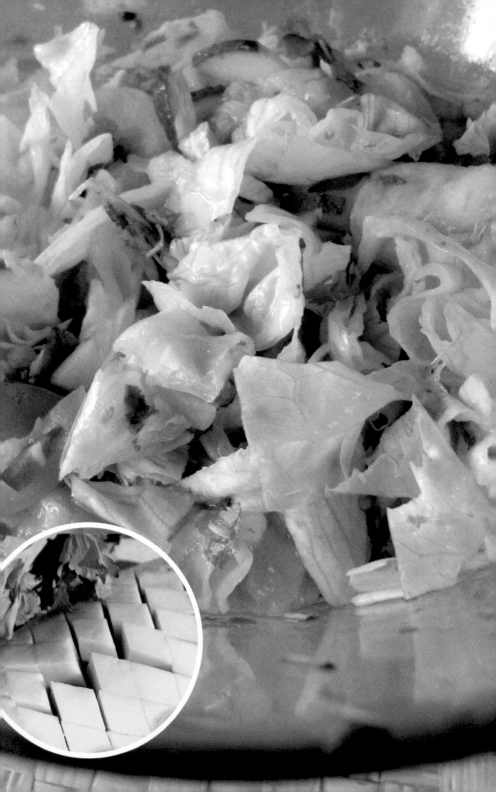

SWEET ICEBERG MIX
With Mango Dressing

- 1/2 head of iceberg lettuce
- 1/2 red bell pepper
- 1 mango
- 1 handful of cilantro
- 10 centimetre of cucumber
- 10 cherry tomatoes

Chop the iceberg lettuce into small crunchy pieces and place in a large bowl. Next, slice the bell pepper into rings, removing the seeds, then cut the rings into smaller pieces. Slice the cucumber then cut the slices into quarters. The cherry tomatoes should also be cut into quarters. Chop the cilantro and mix everything in a bowl. Cut the sides off the mango on each side of the pit so you get two "boats". Use the tip of a knife to carefully slice diagonally in both directions into the fruit of each boat, being careful not to damage the skin. Finally scoop out the mango chunks with a spoon and mix them into the salad so the leaves are covered in juice.

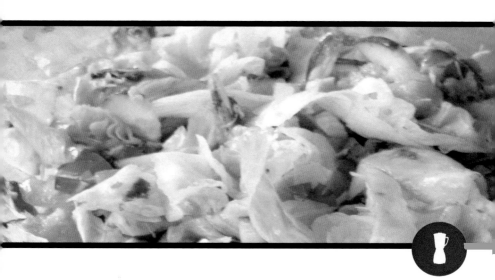

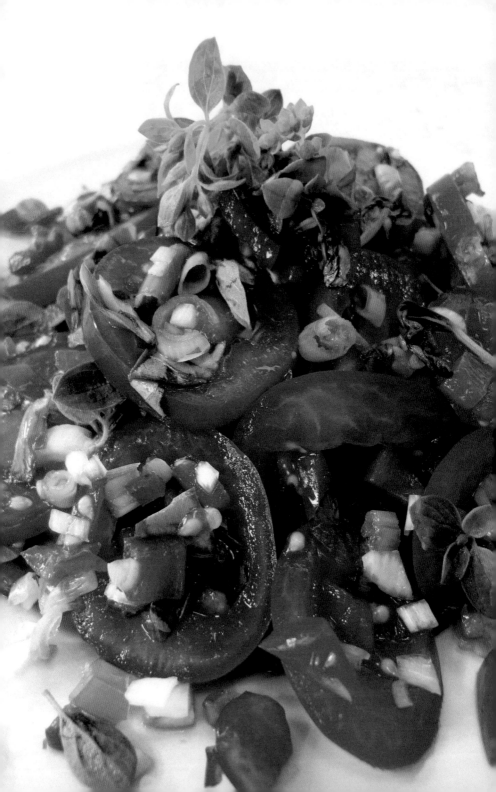

TOMATO SALAD
With Spring Onions

- 8 plum tomatoes
- 1-2 spring onions
- 1 red bell pepper
- 2 stalks of fresh oregano
- 5 leaves of fresh basil
- Optional: lemon juice

Slice the tomatoes and place them in a bowl. Chop the spring onions, the bell pepper, and the fresh herbs in small pieces and mix them in with the tomatoes in the bowl.

Serve the salad on a plate and decorate with some fresh herbs on top. If you like, you can drip juice from a lemon over the top. This salad is great as a side dish, for example as a complement with the sweet falafel.

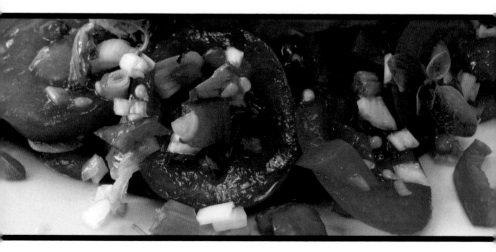

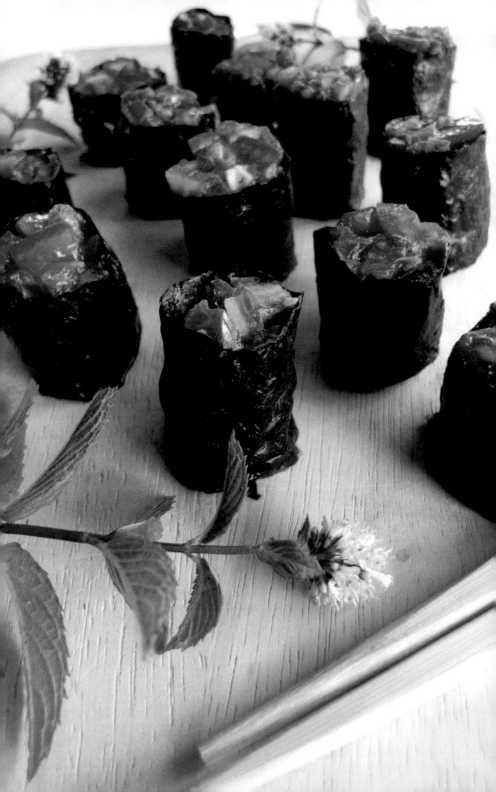

SWEET NORI ROLLS
With Tomatoes and Dates

- 20 small dates
- 3 large plum tomatoes (app. 220 gr)
- 3 sheets of raw nori seaweed

Remove any pits and chop the dates into small pieces. Chop the tomatoes finely and mix dates and tomatoes together in a bowl. Place a nori sheet on a bamboo mat. Use a spoon to spread a 1 to 1 1/2 finger thick line of tomato and date paste at one end of the nori sheet. Roll up the nori sheet using the bamboo mat and close the end with a bit of water using your finger. Lay the rolled nori on a chopping board and slice it into 6 pieces. 3 sheets should make about 18 nori segments in total.

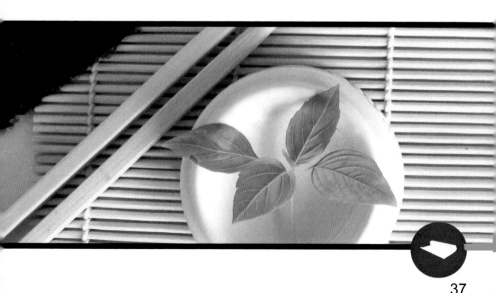

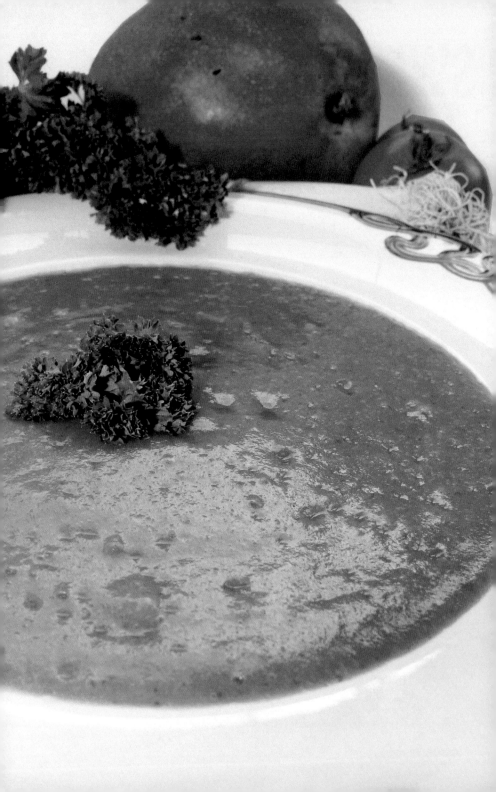

MANGO SOUP
With Parsley

- 2 mangoes
- 4 medium large tomatoes
- 1 spring onion
- 1 sun dried tomato
- 1 handful of parsley
- Optional: water

Separate the fruit pulp or pulp of the mangoes from the large pit and put the mango into a blender along with the fresh tomatoes, the sun dried tomato, the parsley and the spring onion. Blend everything well and add a little water if you want a more liquid soup. Poor the soup into a deep plate and garnish with a sprig of parsley on top.
Serve and enjoy!

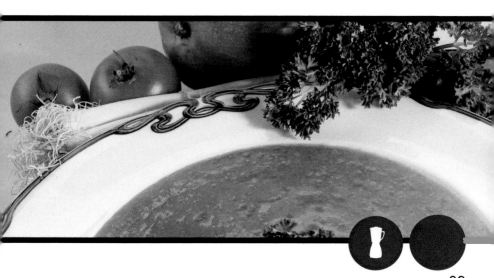

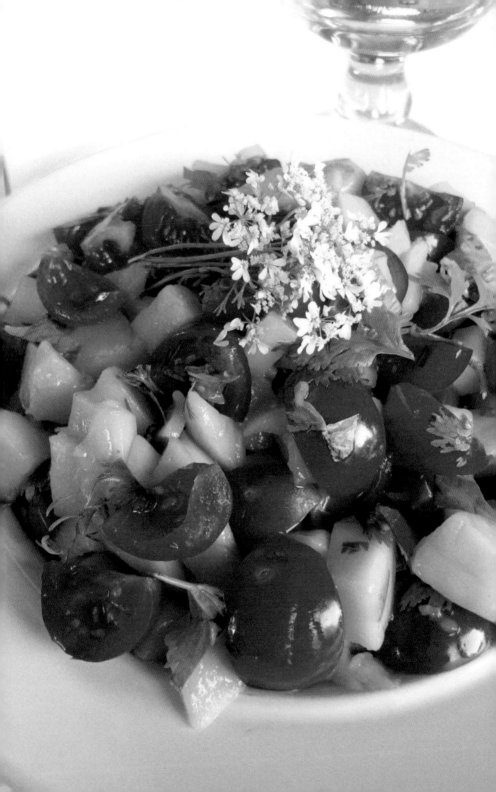

PETR'S MANGO SALAD
With Cilantro

- 2 mangos
- 25 cherry tomatoes
- 1-2 handful of cilantro

This recipe is super simple and super tasty. Slice the fruit pulp from the mangoes into small pieces and cut the tomatoes into quarters. Chop the cilantro (or some other fresh herb of your choice) and mix everything well together. Serve on a plate and decorate with edible flowers.

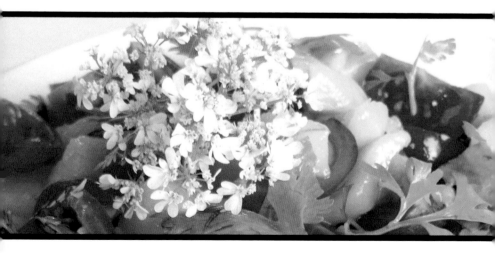

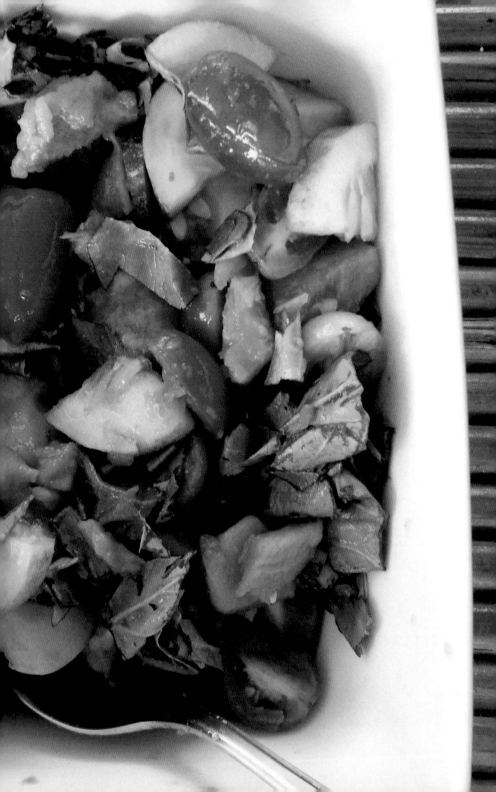

PAPAYA SALAD
With Lemon

- 1/2 cucumber
- 10 cherry tomatoes
- 1 papaya
- 1/2 head of lettuce
- 1/2 lemon

Cut the cucumber into slices and then into quarters. Halve the tomatoes and chop the lettuce. Cut the papaya into half and remove the seeds with a spoon. Use the tip of a knife to carefully slice diagonally in both directions into the fruit pulp of each half but without damaging the skin. Finally scoop out the square papaya dice with a spoon and mix them into the salad. Squeeze the juice from the lemon on top as a dressing.

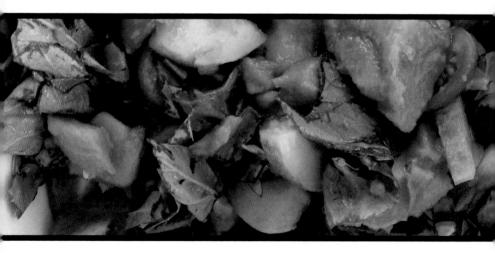

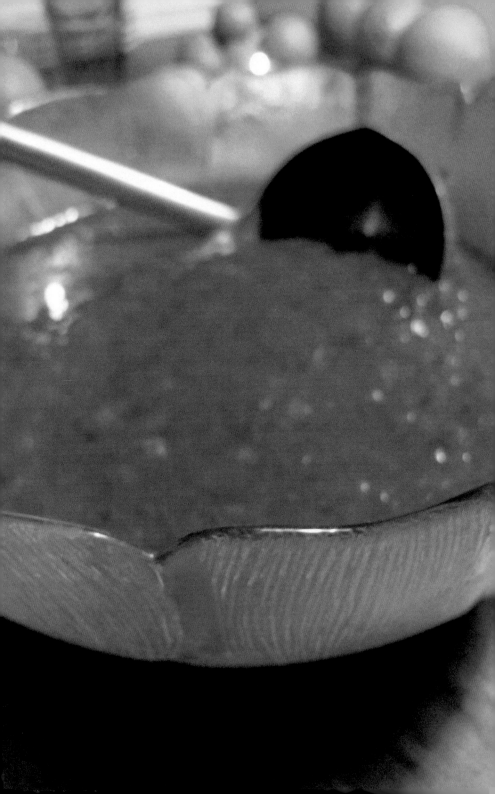

STRAWBERRY DREAM
Sauce, Jam or Soup

- 6 dates
- 6-8 persimmons
- 400 gr fresh or frozen strawberries

This recipe can be used variously as a sauce, a jam, a dip, or a cold soup. Defreeze the strawberries if they are frozen and remove the pit from the dates. Cut the persimmons in halves and blend everything together at a low speed for a short time only. This way you make sure that it is still a bit chunky and has the consistency of home made strawberry jam.

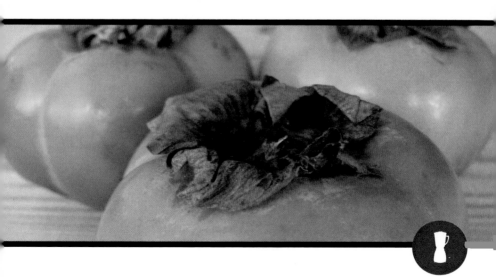

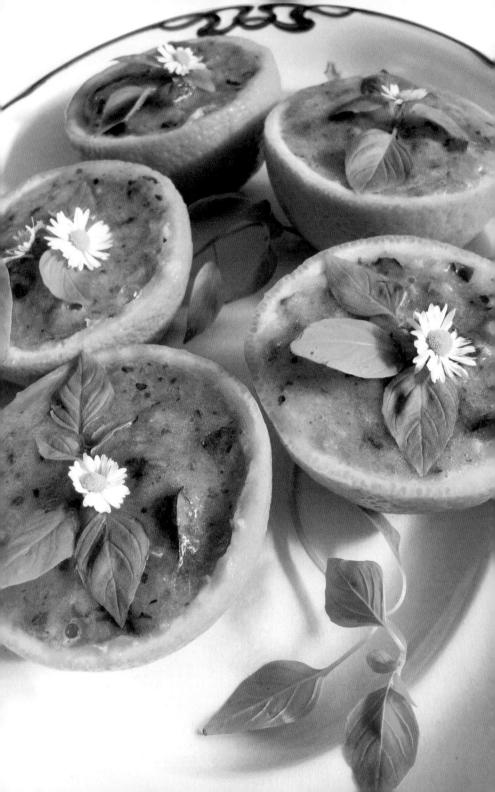

ORANGE DESSERT
With Dates

- 3 oranges
- 20 dates
- 6 daisies
- Some fresh mint or Thai basil for decoration

Cut the oranges into even halves and loosen the fruit pulp carefully from the rind with the tip of a knife. Conserving the rind, carefully remove the fruit pulp with a spoon and cut it into small pieces on a chopping board (remove any seeds in the process). Place the oragne fruit pulp in a bowl and drain some of the juice away if it is very liquid. Remove the pits from the dates and chop the dates into very small pieces. Mix the dates and the oranges carefully together with a spoon until you get a sticky consistency. Next, fill the orange rinds with the paste and decorate them with edible daisies and some mint or Thai-basil on top.

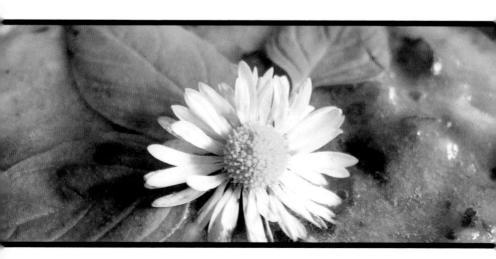

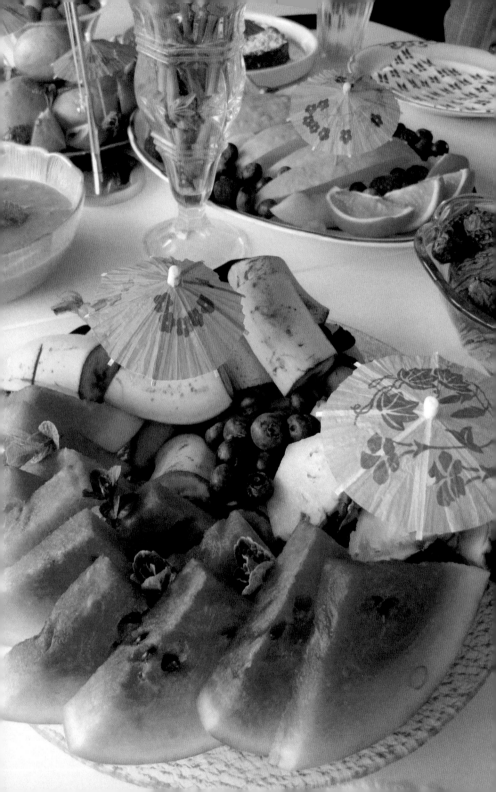

BIRTHDAY IDEAS
For Kids and Adults

- Watermelon
- Honeydew melon
- Bananas
- Pineapple
- Blueberries
- Raspberries
- Strawberries
- Oranges
- Kiwis
- Dates

Be creative for birthdays and celebrations. Slice up pieces of watermelon and honeydew melon and place them on separate platters. Cut a couple of bananas into smaller bits with the skin still attached and place them next to the melons. The same goes for pieces of pineapple. Cut a couple of oranges into quarters and add them to the other platter. Sprinkle different kinds of berries around as decoration and add some festive drinks umbrellas for decoration. Make more platters with for example, kiwi pieces, pitted dates and any other available fruit too. As a centrepiece use the fruit stick recipe on the next page or one of the cakes from this book.

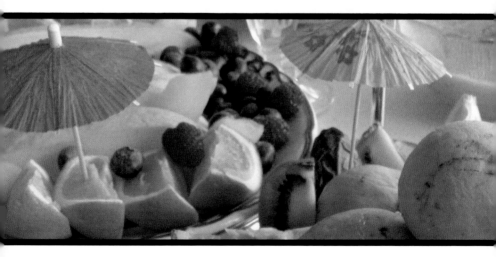

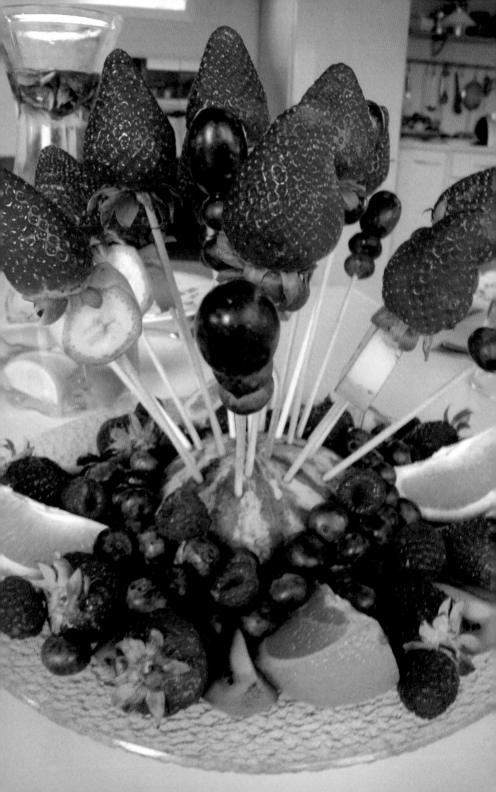

FRUIT STICKS
On a Watermelon Base

- 20 wooden skewer sticks
- 25 fresh strawberries
- 1 banana
- 5-10 grapes
- 1 orange
- 1 watermelon
- 1 kiwi
- 1 cup of blueberries
- 15 raspberries

This is a festive idea for a birthday party. Cut the top off a watermelon and place it face down on a platter (cut up the rest of the watermelon into slices to serve). Wash the fruit but leave the green calix on the strawberries. Without removing the peel, slice the banana into chunks. Skewer various fruits onto the ends of the wooden sticks, like a kebab. For example, a slice of banana and then a strawberry, or two blueberries and a grape. Stick the fruit-kebabs into the watermelon as shown and decorate with various fruit around the base, such as slices of orange, kiwi fruit or berries.

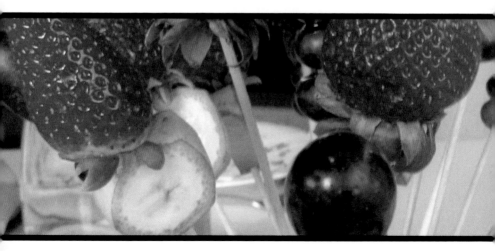

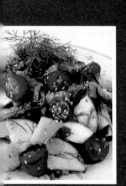 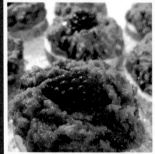 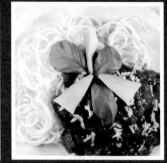 

MEDIUM

Recipes with medium fat content

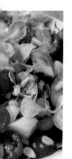
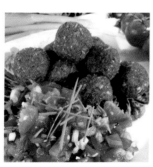
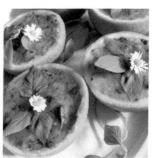
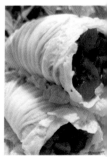

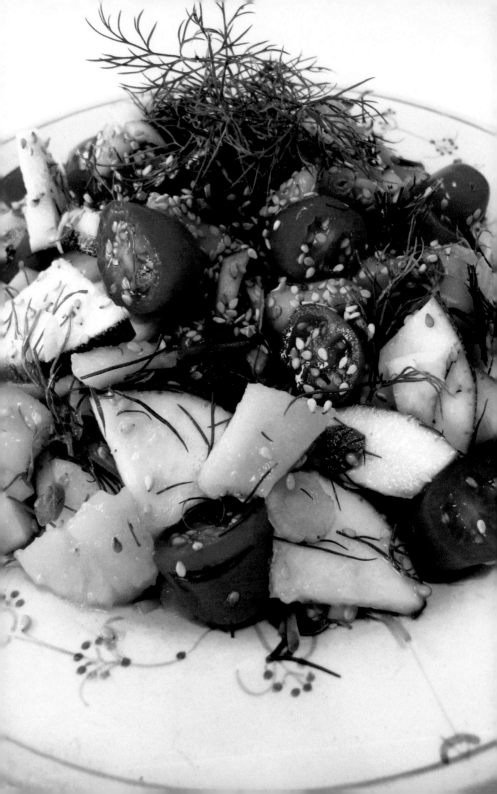

DILL SALAD
Sweet and Sour

- 20 snack tomatoes
- 1 mango
- 1 spring onion
- 1/2 zucchini
- 1 tbsp sesame seeds
- 1 handful of fresh thyme
- 1 handful of fresh dill
- 1/2 lemon

Cut the snack tomatoes into halves and place them in a bowl. Cut the fruit pulp from the mango into smaller pieces and add it to the bowl too. Chop up the spring onion, the thyme, the dill and the zucchini. Mix everything well together along with the sesame seeds. Place the salad on a plate and squeeze the juice of 1/2 lemon over the salad. Finally sprinkle the dish with sesame seeds and garnish with dill.

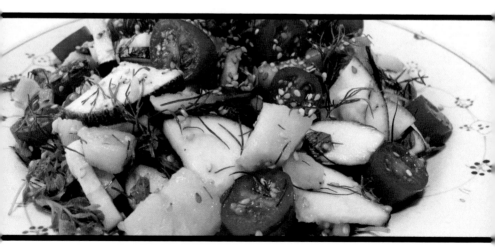

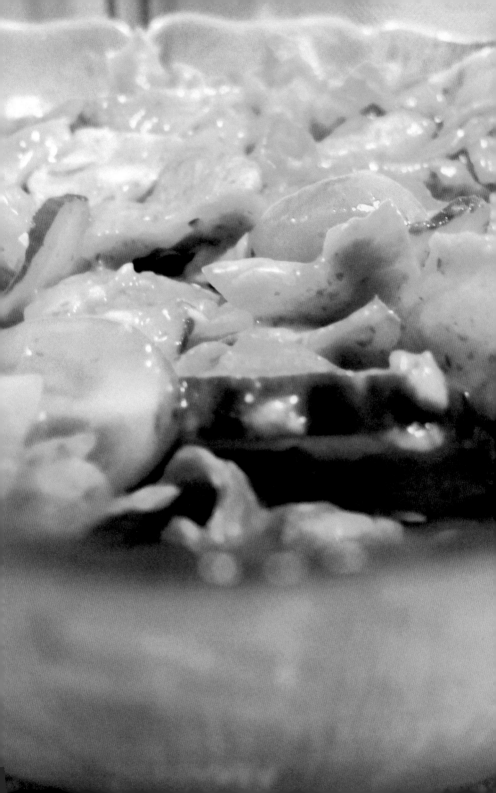

CRUNCHY SALAD
With Mango Dressing

Salad:

- 15 yellow cherry tomatoes
- 100 gr mushrooms
- 1/2 cucumber
- 4 leaves of iceberg lettuce
- Optional: 1 tbsp pine nuts or 1/2 avocado

Dressing:

- 2 mangoes
- 1 handful of fresh cilantro
- 1/2 lime
- 2 ramsons leafs

The salad:

Cut the cherry tomatoes into halves and slice the mushrooms. Dice the cucumber and chop the lettuce a bit too. If you would like something a little more substantial in this salad you can add either pine nuts or avocado. Toss well together in a bowl.

The dressing:

Make the dressing by blending together the fruit pulp of 2 mangoes, the ramsons, the cilantro and the juice of 1/2 a lime into a creamy dressing. Add a little water if needed.

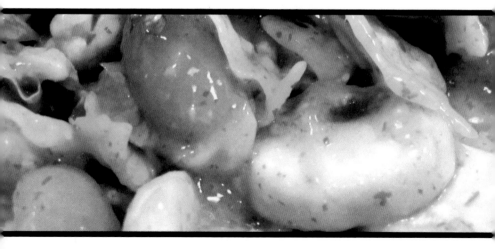

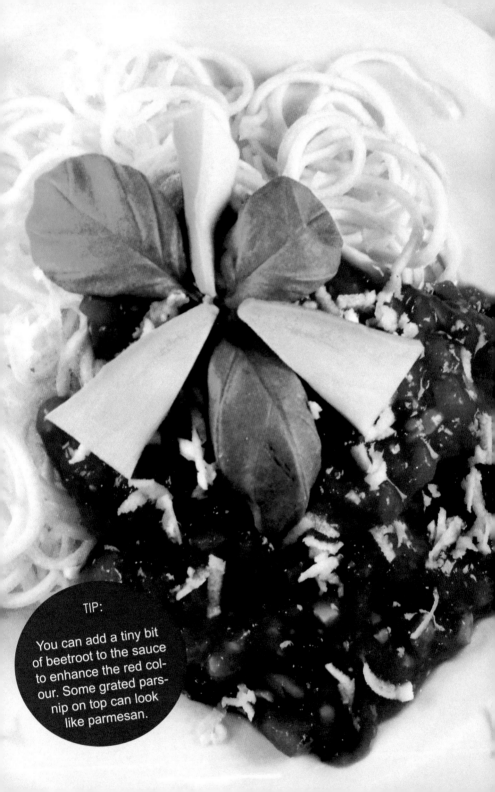

TIP:

You can add a tiny bit of beetroot to the sauce to enhance the red colour. Some grated parsnip on top can look like parmesan.

SPAGHETTI COURGETTE
With Tomato Sauce

- 500 gr red tomatoes
- 10 gr sun dried tomatoes
- 1 mango
- 2-3 small spring onions
- 1 red bell pepper
- 1 zucchini
- 8 leaves of fresh basil
- 4 sprigs of fresh oregano
- 1 tsp pine nuts
- Optional: corn kernels from 1/2 a fresh corn cob
- Optional: 3 mushrooms
- Optional: 1/2 clove of garlic

The spaghetti: Peel the green skin from the zucchini. Use a spiralizer to make long thin noodles or alternatively a julienne peeler.

The sauce: Blend 2/3 of the tomatoes along with the sun dried tomatoes, the mango and optionally, the garlic if you are healthy enough. Blend at high speed into a smooth sauce. Roughly chop the remaining tomatoes, the bell pepper, the spring onions, the basil and the oregano into large pieces and add them to the blender jug along with the pine nuts. (Optionally add some fresh corn or mushrooms too). Blend everything at the lowest setting for a very short time so the sauce remains chunky. Serve and eat right away.

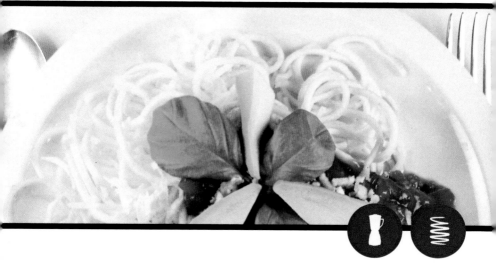

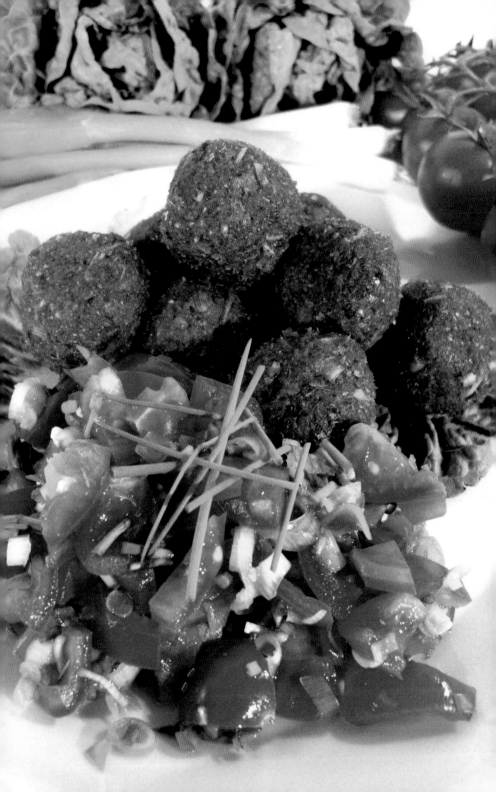

SWEET FALAFEL

With Parsley and Spring Onions

Falafel:

- 7 large dates
- 40 gr flax seeds
- 1 spring onion
- 10 gr cilantro
- 10 gr parsley
- 2 leaves of romaine lettuce

Tomato salad:

- 4 cherry or plum tomatoes
- 1 spring onion
- 6 leaves of chive

Falafel: Grind the flax seeds into a powder in a coffee grinder. Remove the pits from the dates. Add the flax seed powder, the dates, the spring onions, the cilantro and the parsley to a food processor and mix until you have a sticky 'dough'. Shape the dough with your hands into little balls and place them on the romaine lettuce on a plate.

Tomato salad: Finely chop the tomatoes, the spring onion and the chives and mix into a tomato salad (or use the 'Tomato Salad' recipe in this book). Garnish with chives and serve with the falafel.

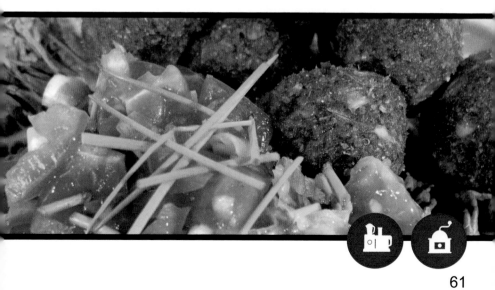

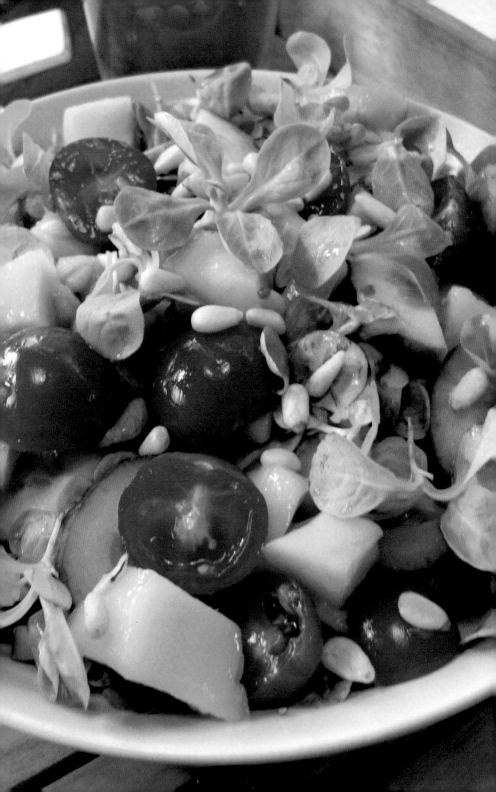

LOUISE'S FAVOURITE
With Mango

- 1/2 cucumber
- 12 cherry tomatoes
- 1-2 handfuld of nut lettuce (Mache)
- 1 mango
- 1 tbsp. pine nuts
- 1/2 lemon

Wash the mâche and place in a bowl. Halve the tomatoes and cut the cucumber into slices and then quarters and add to the salad. Cut off the sides of the mango as close to the pit as you can so you get two 'boats'. Use the tip of a knife to carefully slice diagonally in both directions into the fruit pulp of each boat but without damaging the skin. Finally scoop out the little mango dice with a spoon and mix them in the salad too. Sprinkle the pine nuts on top and finally, squeeze the lemon juice over as a dressing.

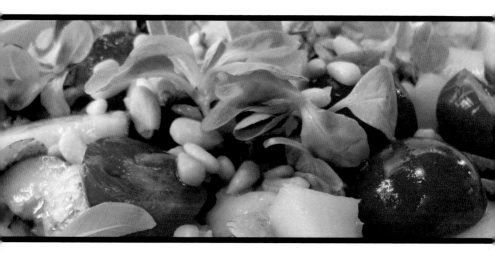

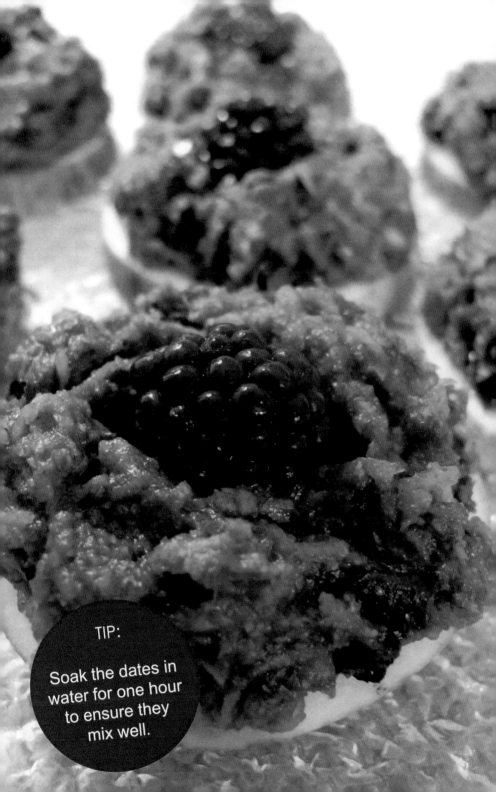

TIP:

Soak the dates in water for one hour to ensure they mix well.

CINNAMON CAKES
On Apple Slices

- 4 medium size carrots
- 22 dates
- 1 cup of blue berries
- 4 tbsp of flax seeds
- 1-2 tsp cinnamon
- 12 fresh blackberries
- 2 apples
-

Peel the carrots and grate them on a very small sized grater into a bowl. Chop the pitted dates and the blueberries into very small pieces on a chopping board and add them to the bowl. Grind up the flax seeds in a coffee grinder and add this to the bowl too along with the cinnamon. Mix everything together well to form a sticky paste using either a fork or a food processor. Then slice the apples into 1cm thick rounds and remove the core with the tip of a knife. Place some paste on each apple slice (not in the middle) and finish by placing a large blackberry in the middle. This recipe will make approximately 10-12 little cakes.

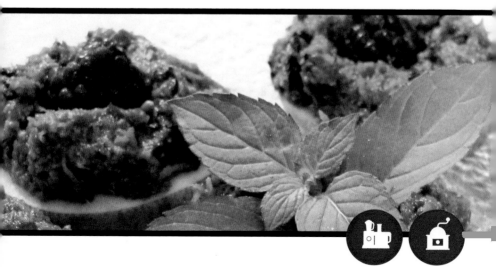

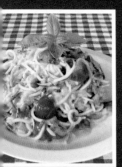
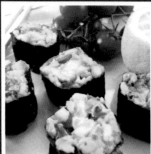
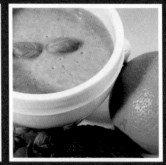

HIGH

Recipes with high fat content

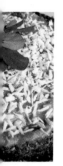 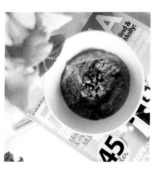 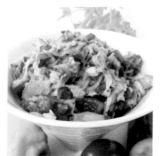 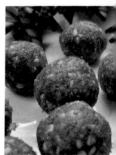

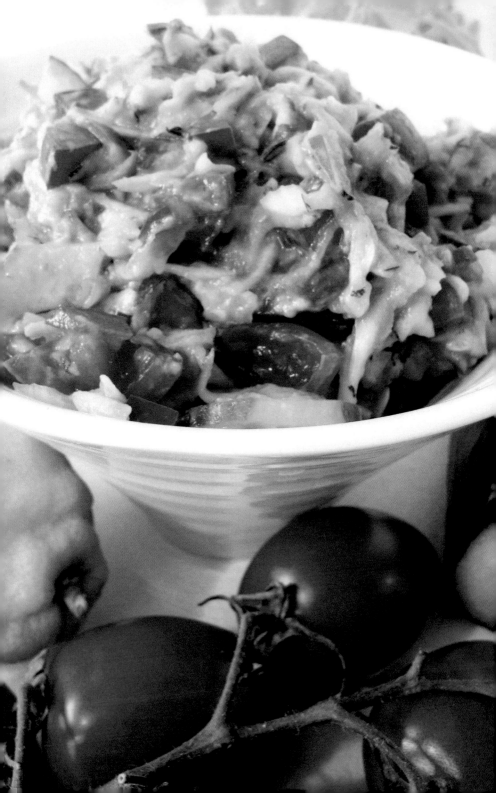

ZUCCHINI SALAD
With Avocado

- 1/2-1 medium zucchini
- 1 red bell pepper
- 1 spring onion
- 1/2 cucumber
- 4-5 plum tomatoes
- 1 stalk of celery
- 1 avocado
- 1/2 lemon

Grate the zucchini into strips with a broad cutting grater and place in a bowl. Chop the bell pepper, the spring onion, the tomatoes, the cucumber and the celery into small pieces and mix with the zucchini strips. Cut the avocado in half and remove the pit. Scoop out the avocado fruit pulp with a spoon and chop it into smaller pieces on a chopping board. Lightly mix the avocado and the juice of 1/2 a lemon into rest of the salad. Serve and enjoy.

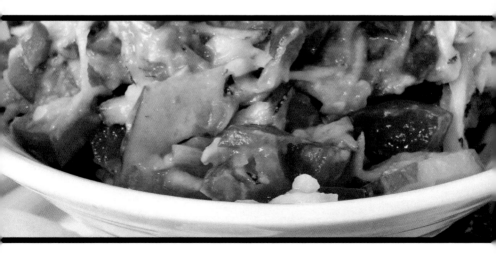

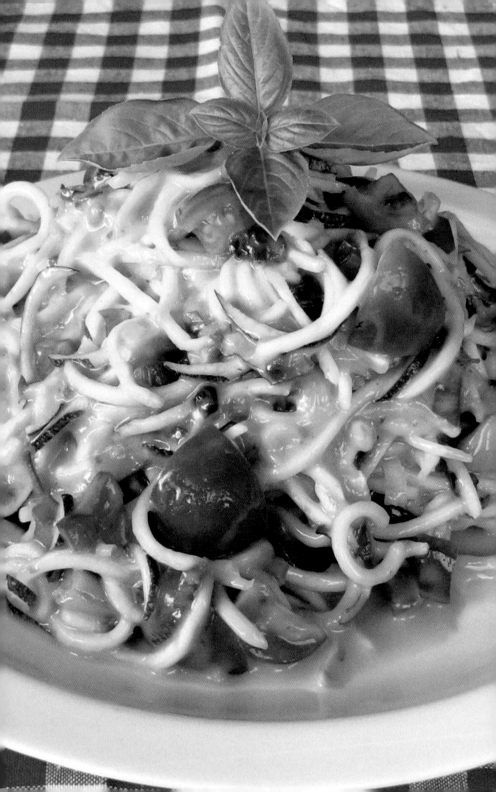

CREAMY 'PASTA'
Italian Style

- 2 zucchini
- 1 avocado
- 2 brown coconuts
- 1 pinch of grated nutmeg
- 1/2 large red bell pepper
- 1 sun dried tomato
- 10 sugar snap peas
- 4 cherry tomatoes
- 1 handful of fresh basil

Prepare in advance by soaking the sun dried tomatoes in water for 1 hour. Pour the milk from the two coconuts into a blender and add the avocado and a pinch of grated nutmeg. Add some of the coconut flesh (chopped) to the milk as well. Blend into a creamy sauce then pour it into a bowl. Use a spiralizer or a julienne peeler to make long noodle look-alike strips from the zucchini. Toss the zucchini noodles with the sauce. Prepare the rest of the ingredients as follows: Chop the bell pepper into little squares and the sun dried tomato into very small pieces. Cut each sugar snap pea into four and the fresh tomatoes into quarters. Roughly chop the fresh basil. Add all of it to the sauce and using a fork, mix it all well.

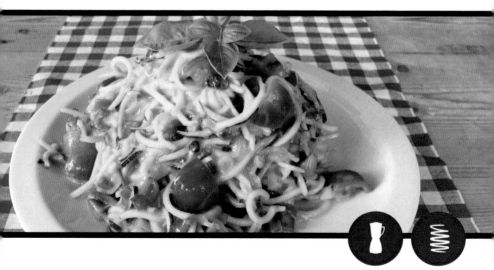

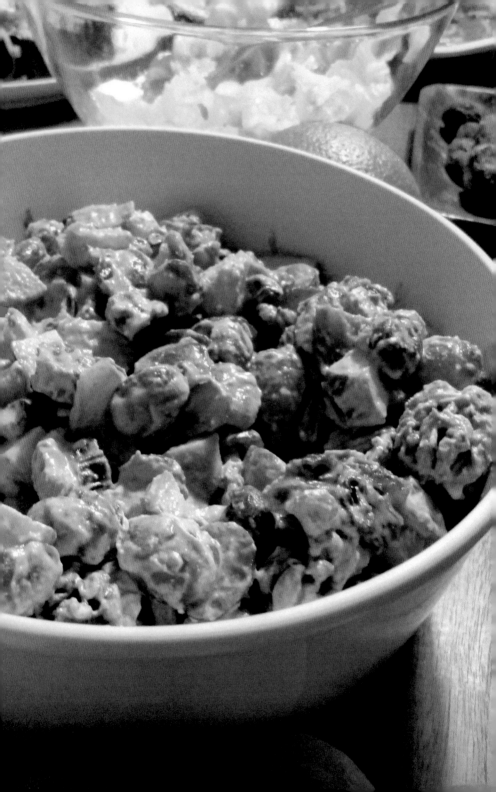

WALDORF SALAD
By Christina Søberg

The salad:
- 3-4 stalks of celery
- 300g grapes
- 2 apples, cored
- 1 dl raisins or dates
- 50g walnuts

The crème:
- 1 dl cashew nuts (60 gr)
- 1-2 oranges
- A pinch of vanilla

Soak the cashew nuts in water for 2 hours.

The salad: Cut the celery and the pitted dates into small pieces (if you use raisins don't chop them). Dice up the apples, first removing the cores. Chop the walnuts into large chunks but save a few for decoration. Cut the grapes into halves and mix everything together in a bowl.

The crème: Drain the soaked cashews and blend in a blender along with the vanilla and 1-2 oranges until you get a creamy consistency. Pour the crème onto the salad and mix well. Decorate with grapes, walnuts and perhaps some grated orange peel.

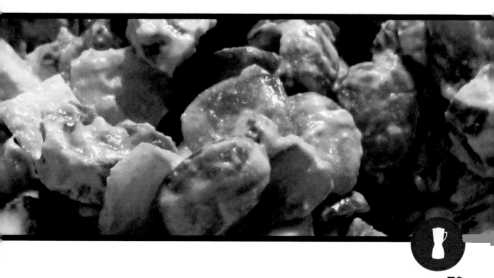

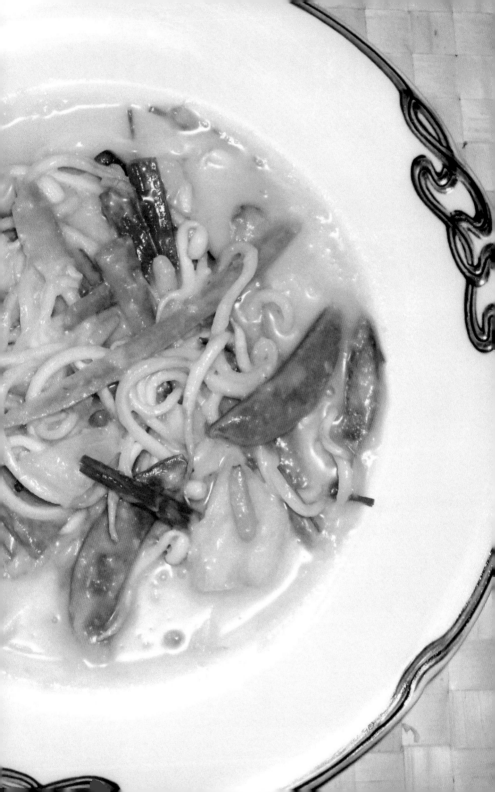

THAI NOODLES
With Coconut Sauce

- 1 zucchini
- 1 fresh young coconut
- 2 mandarins or 1 orange
- 1 slice of pineapple
- 1/2 red bell pepper
- 1 spring onion
- 1 carrot
- 2 handfuls of bean sprouts
- 10-15 sugar snap peas
- 3 sprigs of cilantro
- Optional: 1/2 clove of garlic
- Optional: a pinch of chilli

Noodles: Peel the zucchini and slice it into noodles with a spiralizer or julienne peeler. Place the zucchini noodles in a large bowl.

The sauce: Remove the pulp from the young green coconut and blend together with the water and mandarins (or orange). If you are fairly healthy you can add some garlic or chilli to the blender. Pour the sauce over the noodles. Slice the bell pepper, the spring onion and the carrot into long thin pieces. Cut the pineapple into little squares, roughly chop the cilantro and add it all to the bowl. Add the sugar snap peas and the bean sprouts and fold all together well.

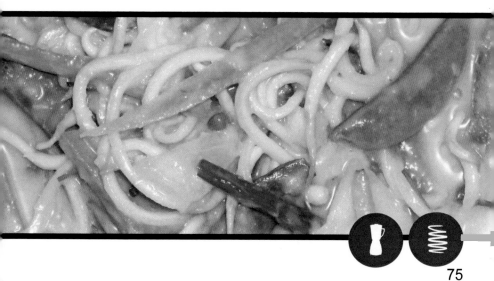

75

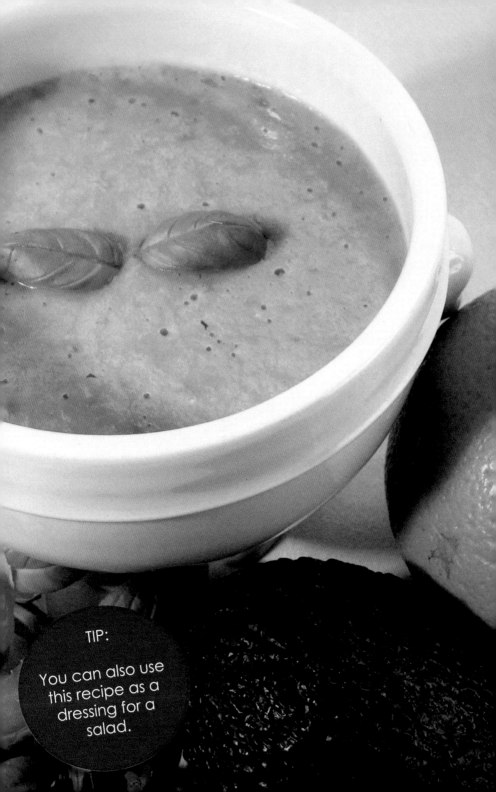

TIP:

You can also use this recipe as a dressing for a salad.

ORANGE SOUP
With Fresh Herbs

- 2 oranges
- 1 avocado
- 1 handful of fresh thyme or basil

Peel the oranges and remove the seeds. Remove the fruit pulp from the avocado and put the oranges and the avocado into a blender. Add a handful of fresh thyme or basil according to what you like the most. Blend everything well into a creamy, sweet and delicious soup. If you have a powerful blender like a Vitamix or Blendtech you can blend for a little while so it becomes a bit lukewarm. Serve in a soup plate and garnish with fresh herbs.

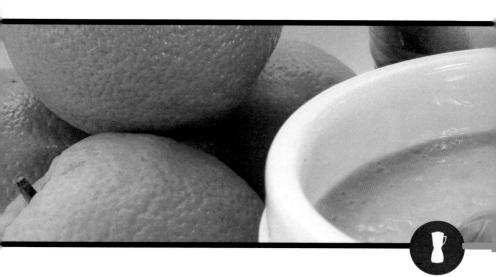

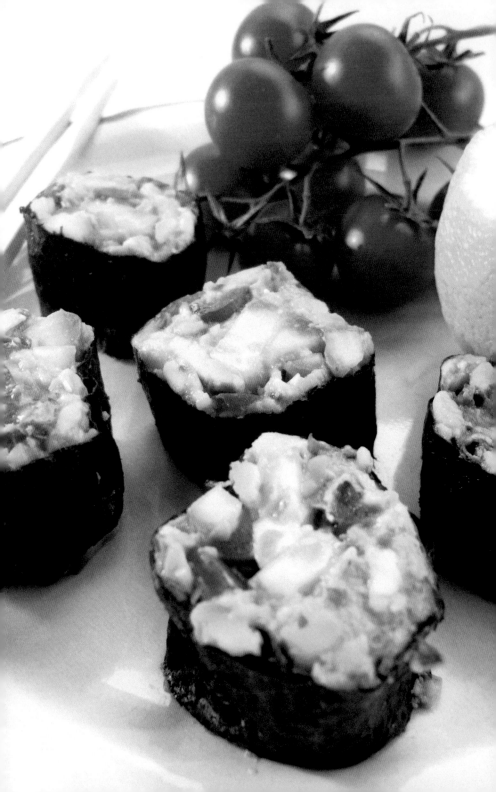

AVOCADO MAKI
With Pine Nuts

- 2 avocados
- 7 cherry tomatoes
- 4 cm cucumber
- 6 baby spinach leaves
- 1 spring onion
- 2 tsp pine nuts
- 1 tsp sesame seeds
- 1/2 lemon
- 2-3 sheets of raw nori seaweed

Chop the cherry tomatoes, the spring onion and the baby spinach into small pieces. Place them in a bowl and add the pine nuts and sesame seeds. Remove the fruit pulp from the avocado and add to the bowl along with the lemon juice and mix everything together well with a spoon or fork to form a chunky paste. Place a nori sheet on a bamboo mat. Use a spoon to spread a 2 finger thick line of the paste at only one end of the nori sheet. Cut the cucumber into long thin slices and place a line of cucumber on top. Roll up the nori sheet with the bamboo mat and close the end with a bit of water using your finger. Place the rolled up nori on a chopping board and cut it into approx. 3 or 4 cm long segments with a very sharp knife.

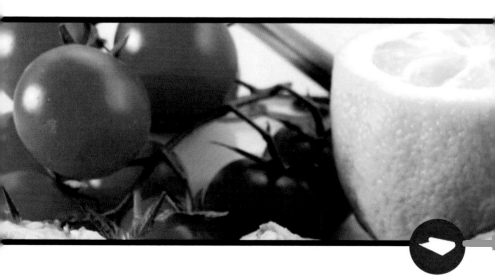

79

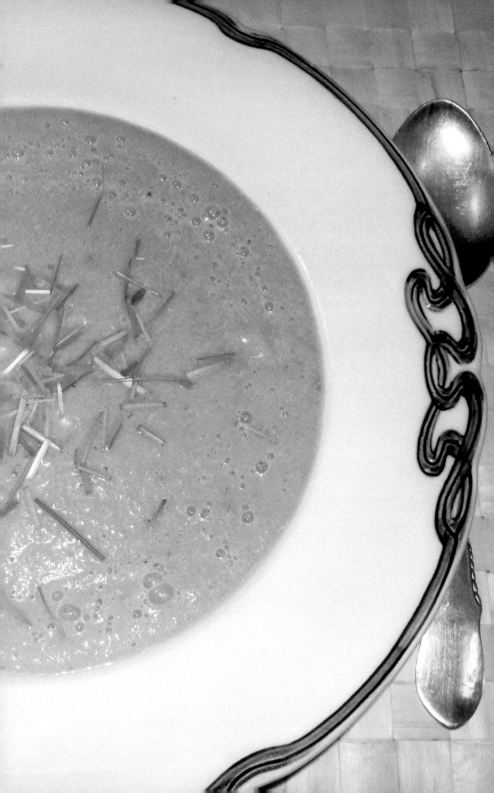

ASPARAGUS SOUP
With Avocado

- 15-20 asparagus
- 1 avocado
- 1/2 cucumber
- 1/2 lemon
- 1 tbsp pine nuts
- A pinch of grated nutmeg
- A little bit of chives or dill
- 1/2 glass of water

Cut the asparagus and the cucumber into small chunks and put them into a blender along with the fruit pulp from the avocado. Remove the peel and the seeds from 1/2 a lemon and add the lemon as well. Add a tbsp of pine nuts, a pinch of grated nutmeg and approx 1/2 glass of water. Blend everything into a creamy soup, adding more water if it is too thick. Pour the soup into a deep plate and decorate with either chives or dill. Serve and enjoy.

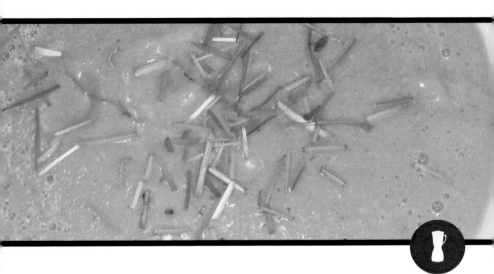

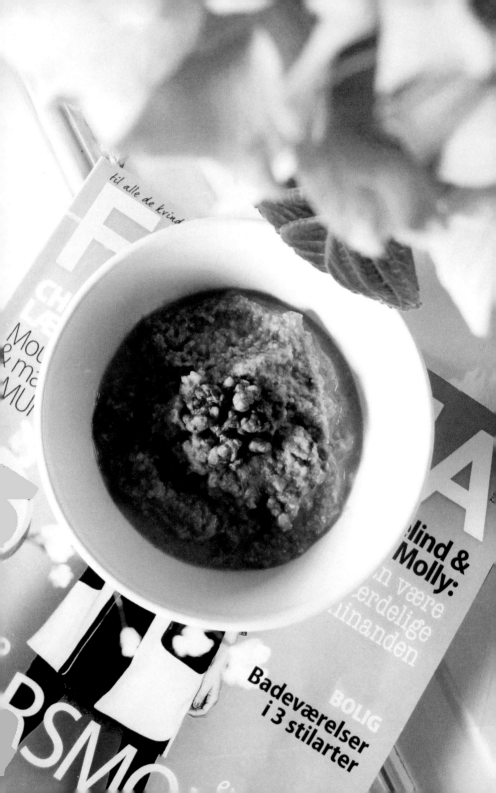

WALNUT DIP
With Jerusalem Artichokes

Sticks:

- 1/2 zucchini
- 2 stalk of celery
- 2 carrots

Dip:

- 4-6 Jerusalem artichokes
- 10 gr pine nuts
- 20 gr walnuts
- 1 sun dried tomato
- 1-2 dl water

Sticks: Cut some long sticks of zucchini, celery and carrots and stand them in glasses.

Dip: Wash the Jerusalem artichokes carefully and chop them into small chunks. Add the artichokes, the pine nuts, the walnuts, the sun dried tomato and 1 or 2 dl of water into a food processor or a strong blender. Mix everything into a creamy paté. Serve the dip in a small bowl next to the sticks and eat right away.(This dish tends to separate from the dip when left to stand).

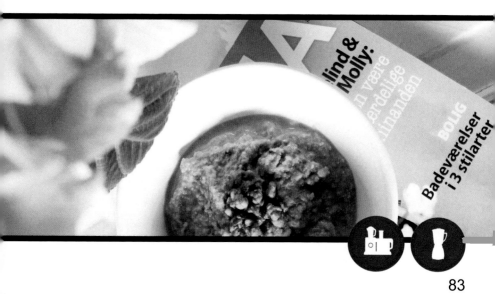

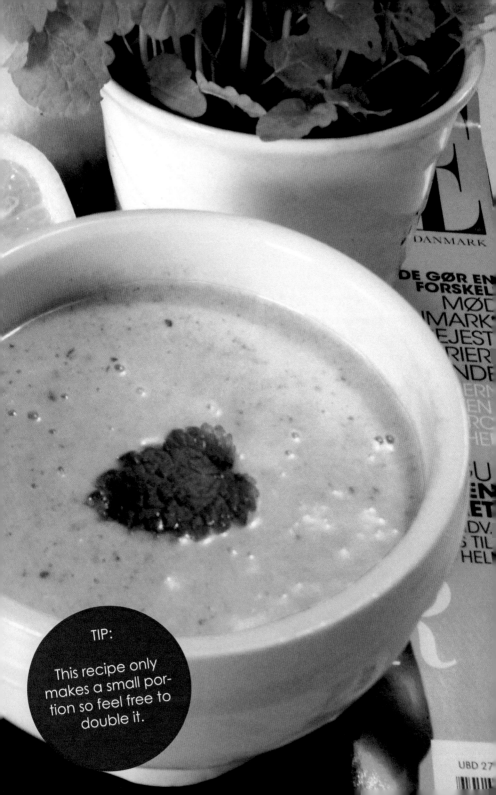

TIP:

This recipe only makes a small portion so feel free to double it.

COCONUT SOUP
With Sesame and Lemon

- 1 young fresh coconut
- 1/2 lemon
- 2 tbsp of sesame seeds
- 1/3 spring onion
- 1-2 dates
- 7 leafs of lemon balm
- Optional: water

Grind the sesame seeds into a powder in a coffee grinder. Take the fruit pulp and the coconut water from a fresh young coconut and put it into the blender. Add the ground up sesame seeds, the lemon balm leaves, the juice of 1/2 a lemon, the pitted dates and 1/3 of a spring onion to the blender as well. Blend everything well until you get a creamy soup and add more water if you find it too thick. Decorate with a few lemon balm leaves on top and enjoy.

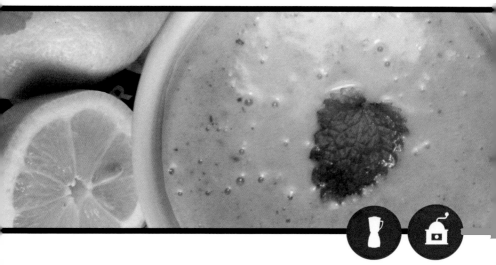

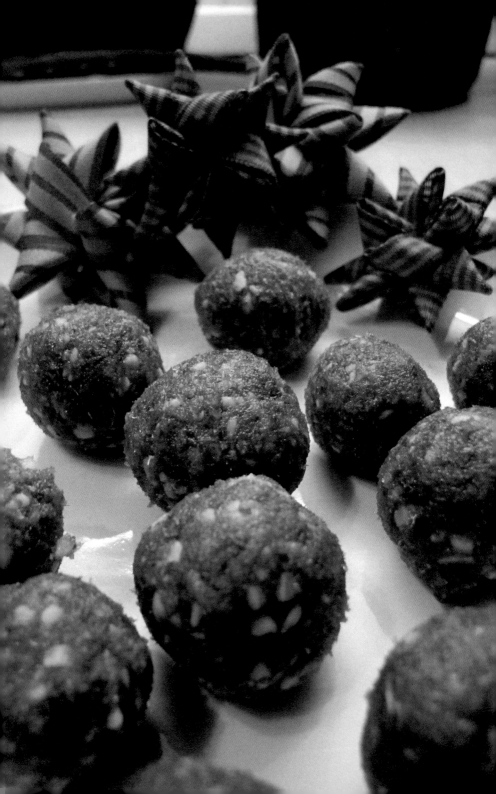

CHRISTMAS COOKIES
By Sandra Holm

- 600 gr dates
- 1 dl almonds (50 gr)
- 1 tsp ground up cloves
- 1 tsp ground up cinnamon
- 1 pinch ground up ginger

Place the almonds in a food processor and grind them into a crunchy powder. Add the ground cloves, cinnamon and ginger. Remove the pits from the dates and add them to the food processor and mix all together until you get a fairly even paste. Use your hands to roll the paste into small balls and place them on a platter. Serve and enjoy.

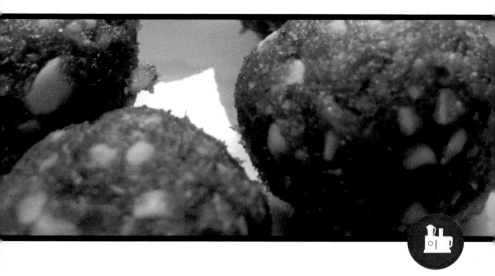

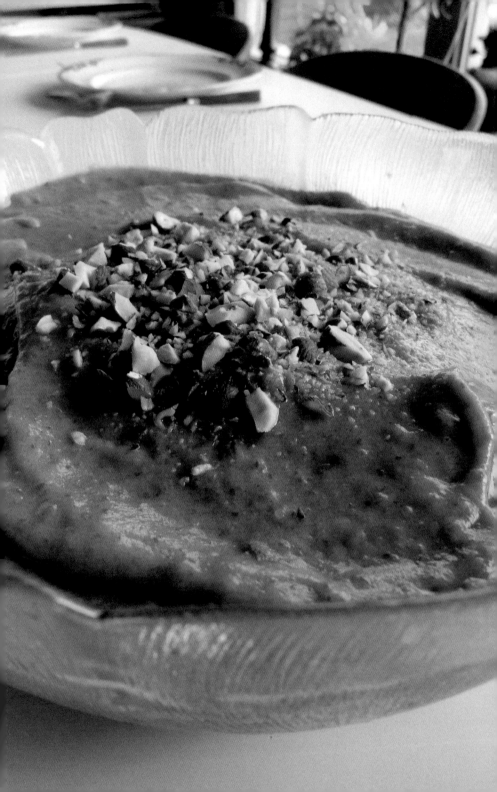

DANISH APPLE 'PIE'
With Cinnamon

The crème:

- 14 Medjoul dates
- 2 small glasses of water
- 1 tsp. ground up cinnamon
- 1 pinch of ground up vanilla

Layering:

- 8-10 bananas
- 6 apples
- 70 gr hazel nuts

Crème: Blend the dates (pitted) water, cinnamon and vanilla to a thick creme in a blender.

Layers: Peel and core the apples, then grate them on a grater using the largest cutter. Peel the bananas and slice them horizontally into long slices. Roughly chop the hazel nuts into small pieces, conserving some for decoration. Take a large bowl and place the ingredients in layers in the following order:

1. Slices of banana
2. Grated apple
3. The date crème
4. Sprinkle with hazel nuts
5. Slices of banana
6. Grated apple
7. A thin layer of date crème on the top
8. Decorate with the rest of the hazel nuts

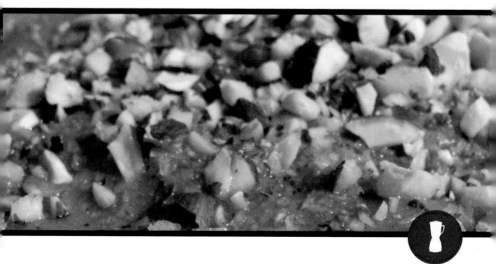

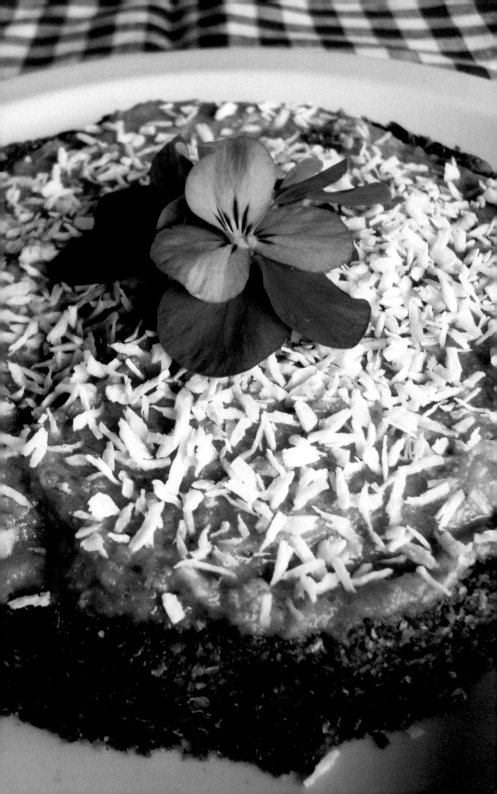

COCONUT CAKE
With Orange Crème

Crust:
- 6 dates
- 65 gr flax seed

Crème:
- 6 dates
- 1 orange
- 30 gr flaxseed
- 1-2 carrots
- 2 tbsp shredded coconut
- An edible flower
- Optional: water

The crust: Grind the flax seeds into a powder in a coffee grinder. Put the pitted dates and the flax seed powder into a food processor and mix to form a sticky paste. Spread the paste onto a flan dish and press out with your fingers to form a crust with high edges.

The creme: Grate the carrots on a grater, and grind the flax seeds in a coffee grinder. Place into a food processor: the pitted dates; the peeled orange; the ground flax seeds; the grated carrots and most of the shredded coconut. Mix into a thick crème, adding a tiny bit of water if needed. Pour the crème onto the crust and decorate with the rest of the shredded coconut and as a suggestion, garnish with edible violets.

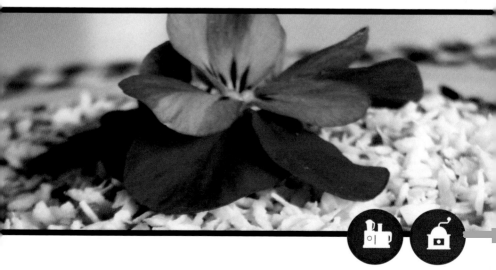

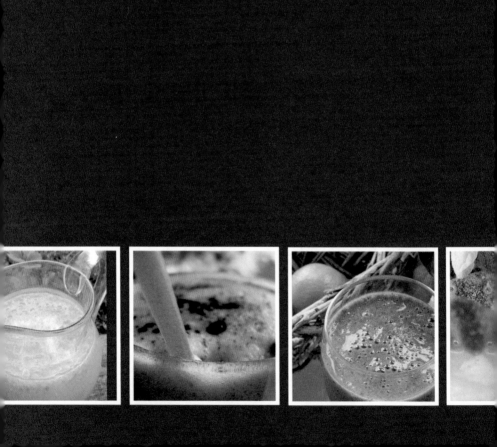

DRINKS

Juices and smoothies

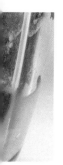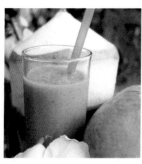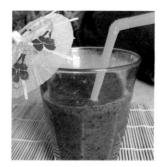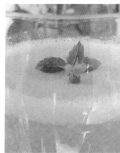

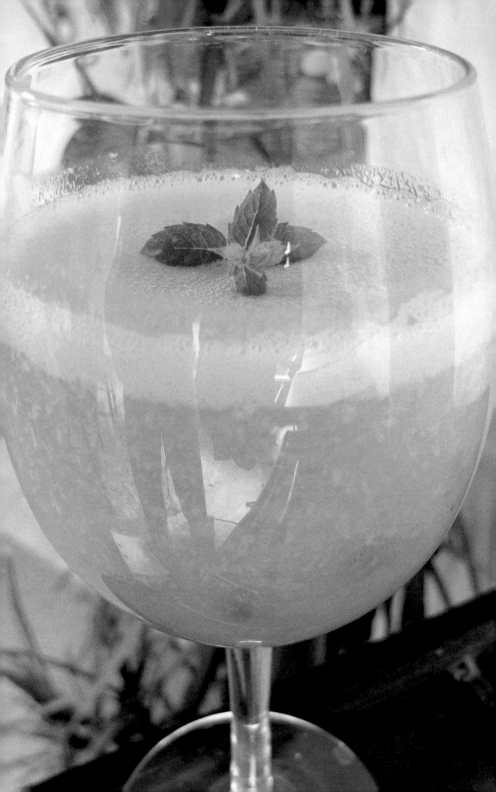

TROPICAL JUICE
With Mango

- 10 sweet oranges
- 1 mango
- 1 passion fruit
- 1 sprig of fresh mint
- Optional: Ice cubes

Juice the oranges with a citrus press or citrus juicer and pour the juice into a blender. Add the fruit pulp from the mango and blend together the mango and the orange juice into a sweet drink. Pour the juice into a jug and add the passionfruit pulp. Stir well and serve in a glass, garnish with some mint leaves. Add ice cubes if you like.

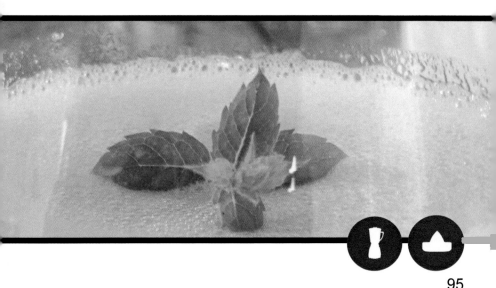

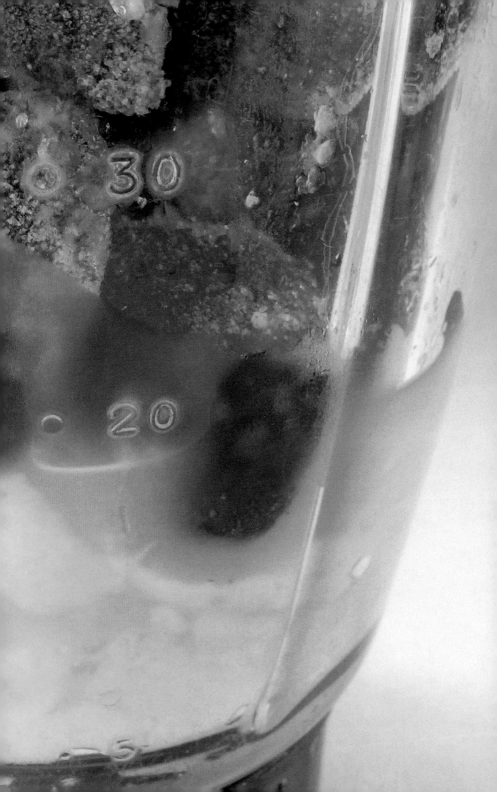

EXOTIC SMOOTHIE
With Strawberries

- 1/3 pineapple
- 2 mangoes
- 10 frozen or fresh strawberries
- 1-2 glasses of water

Put the fruit pulp of 2 mangoes into a blender. Add the chopped pineapple and the strawberries, either frozen or fresh. You can leave the calix (green tops) on the strawberries if you like. Add 1-2 glasses of water to raise the level to about the middle of the blender jug. Blend at a high speed and enjoy a glass of sweet exotic smoothie.

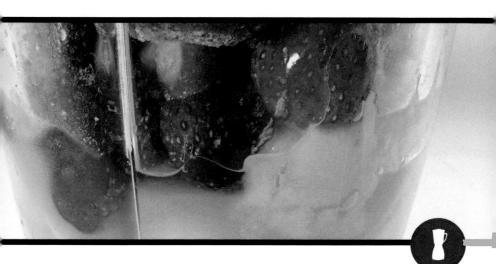

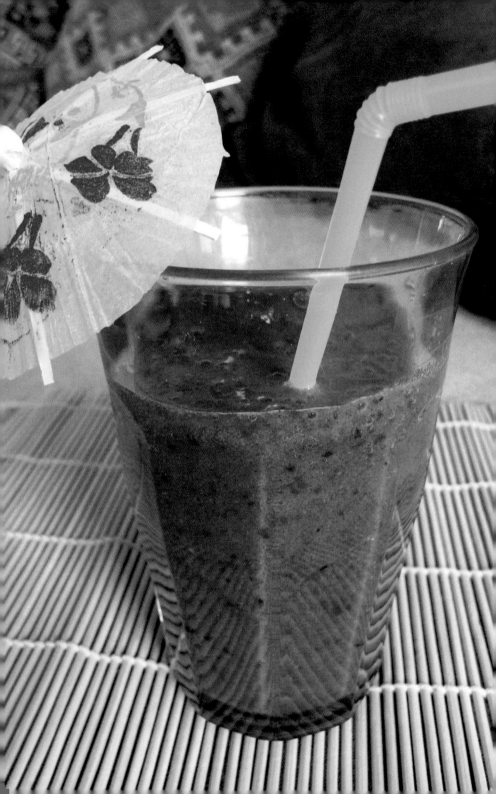

KIDS SMOOTHIE
With Raspberry and Blackberry

- 3 - 4 bananas
- 1 cup of blackberries
- 1 cup of raspberries
- 8-10 dates
- 1-2 glasses of water

Put into a blender, the fresh blackberries and the raspberries (you can use frozen berries if you defrost them a bit in advance). Add the bananas and the pitted dates and pour in 1-2 glasses of water. Blend well, adding more water if you prefer a thinner smoothie. Pour the smoothie into a glass and decorate in a child-friendly and appealing manner as desired.

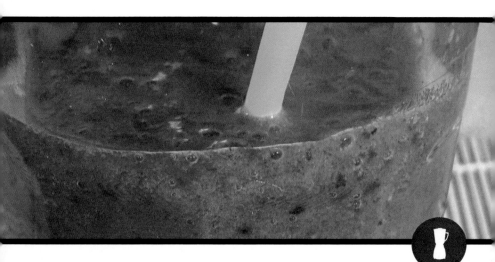

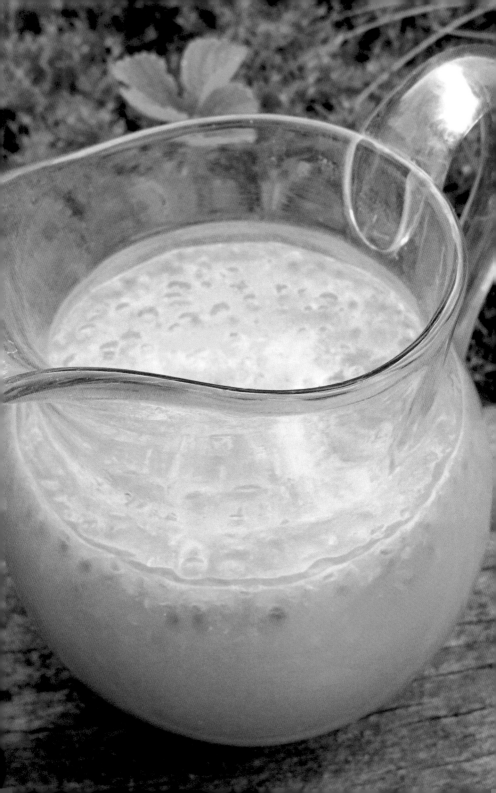

ORANGE JUICE
With Passion Fruit

- 10 oranges
- 2-3 passion fruits
- Optional: ice cubes
-

This drink is as simple and tasty as it gets and you only need two ingredients. Juice the oranges with a citrus juicer and pour into a jug. Cut the passion fruit in half and remove the pulp with a spoon. Add the passion fruit to the freshly squeezed orange juice and stir well. Add ice cubes if you like.

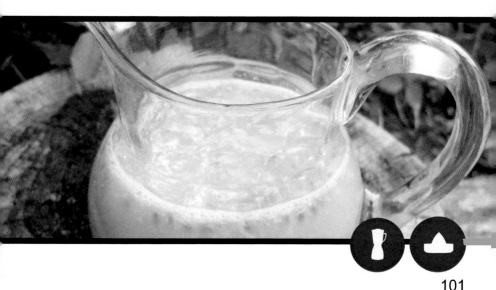

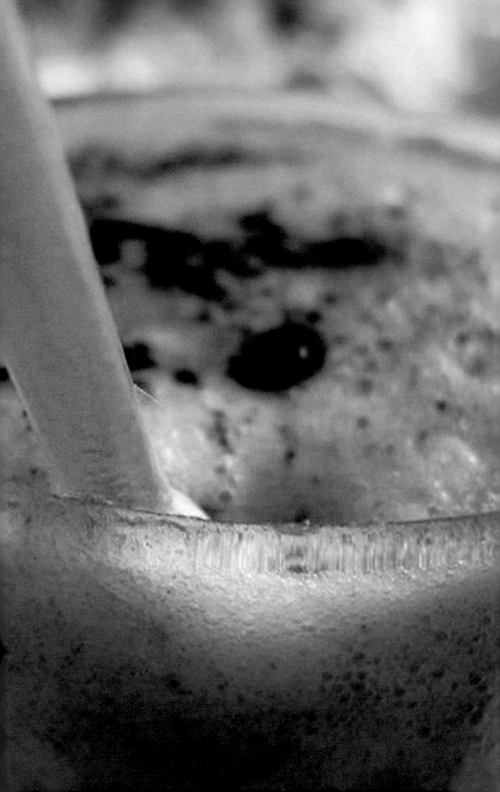

DATORADE
With Cinnamon

- 15 dates
- 1-3 bananas
- 1 tsp cinnamon (or carob or vanilla)
- 3-4 glasses of water

Remove the pits from the dates and put all 15 pitted dates in the blender. Add 1-2 glasses of water and blend at high speed to form an even consistency. Add 1-2 more glasses of water and blend until you get a slightly airy foam on top. Add the bananas and a teaspoon of either cinnamon, carob or vanilla (not cacao) and blend until slightly creamy and smooth. Serve in a cup or glass and sprinkle with carob, cinnamon or vanilla on top. Drink right away.

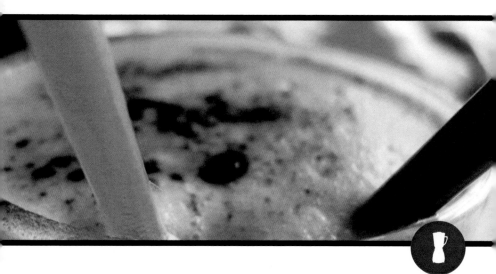

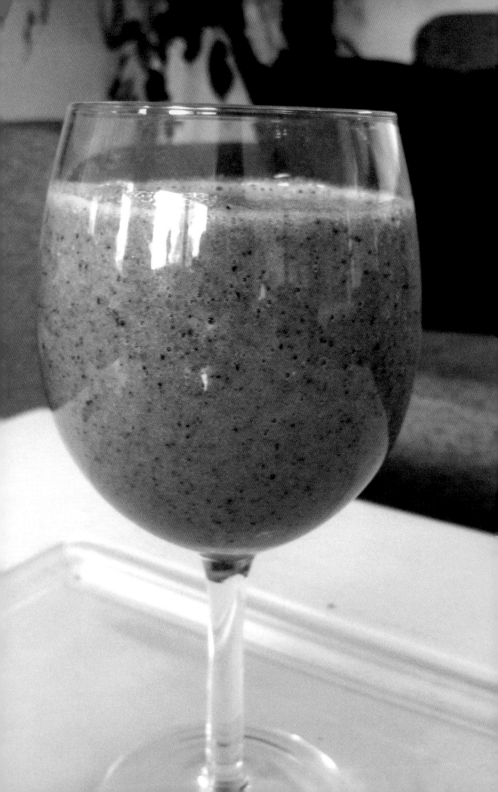

BLUEBERRY SMOOTHIE
With Bananas

- 8 bananas
- 100-150 gr frozen blueberries
- 1-2 cups of water

Sometimes it is super-simple to be healthy and this smoothie is for sure, simple. Firstly, peel the bananas and put all 8 bananas into your blender. Secondly add the frozen blueberries to the blender and pour in the water too. Blend at high speed until you get a creamy smoothie and serve it in a beautiful glass. Enjoy.

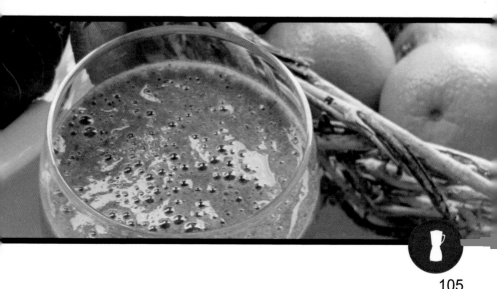

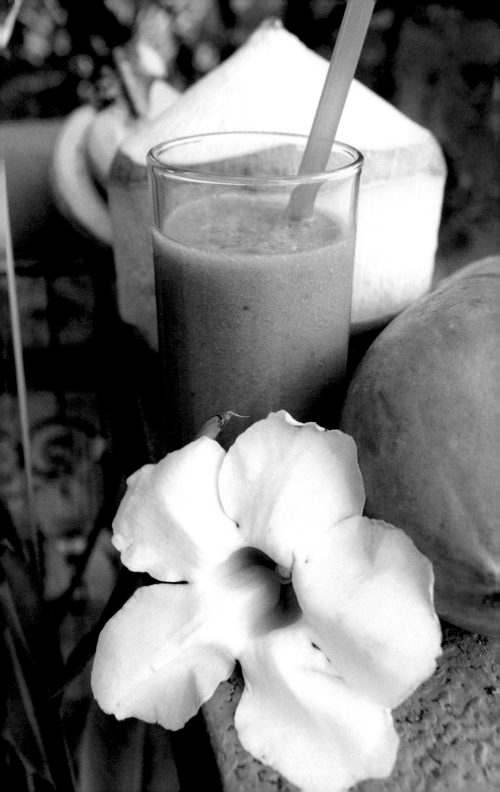

BANANA SMOOTHIE
With Coconut Water

- 7 bananas
- The water from 1 young coconut
- 1 small papaya

Peel the bananas and put them into the blender. Next, cut the papaya in two and remove the seeds with a spoon. Add the ripe papaya fruit pulp to the blender (but not the skin or the seeds). Finally add the water from a young coconut and blend at high speed till you get a creamy delicious smoothie. You can decorate the smoothie glass with a thin slice of pineapple or a slice of orange on the rim. Enjoy.

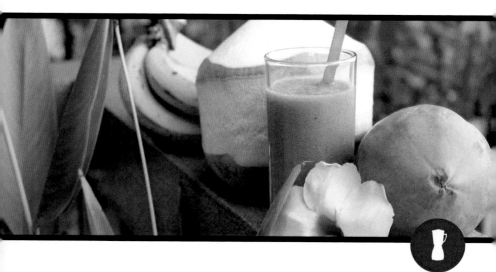

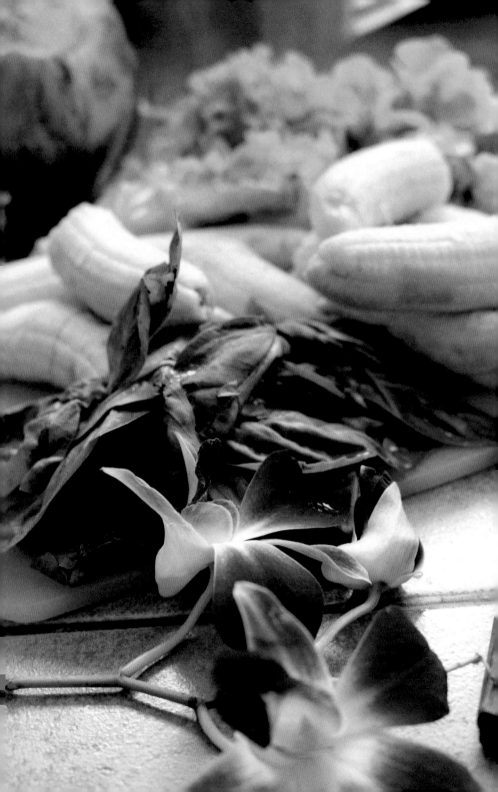

GREEN SMOOTHIE
With Basil

- 1/2 head of soft lettuce
- 7 bananas
- 2 handful of fresh basil
- Optional: 1 fresh young coconut

Rinse the lettuce and the fresh basil carefully. Peel the bananas and put them in the blender. Add the lettuce and the fresh basil. Fill the blender jug to half way with water or optionally, with the coconut water from a fresh young coconut (not creamy coconut milk).

Blend well and serve in a beautiful glass with a flower or a piece of fruit on the rim.

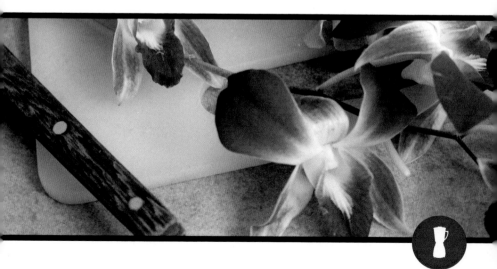

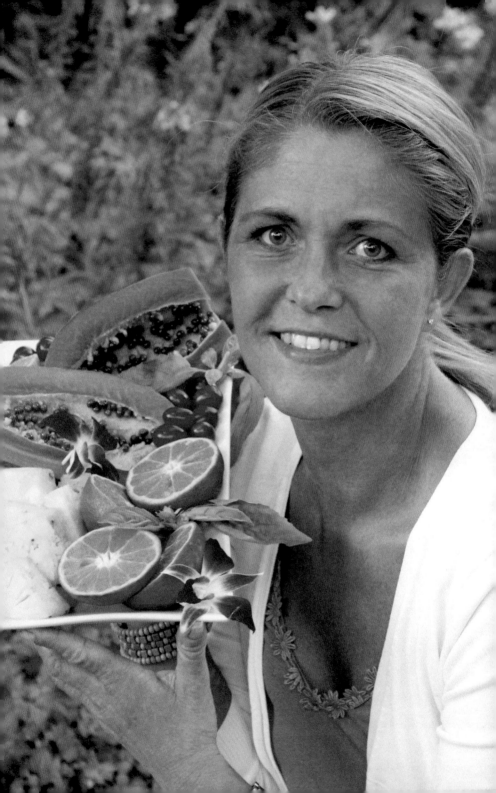